IAFF/IAFC/ACE
PEER FITNESS TRAINER
REFERENCE MANUAL

A Collaborative Effort by:

The International Association of Fire Fighters,

The International Association of Fire Chiefs,

and

The American Council on Exercise

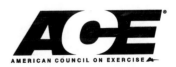

AMERICAN COUNCIL ON EXERCISE

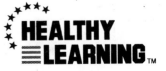

HEALTHY LEARNING™

International Association of Fire Fighters
1750 New York Avenue, NW
Washington, DC 20006
www.iaff.org

Assistant to the General President: Richard M. Duffy
Safety and Health Assistant: Ron McGraw
Project Director: Raymond Wasdyke, Ed.D.
Oversight Committee Chair: Patrick Morrison

Fire Service Joint Labor Management Wellness-Fitness Task Force

IAFF
IAFC
Austin Fire Department, IAFF Local 975
Calgary Fire Department, IAFF Local 255
Charlotte Fire Department, IAFF Local 660
Fairfax County Fire & Rescue Department, IAFF Local 2068

Indianapolis, IN, IAFF Local 416
Los Angeles County Fire Department, IAFF Local 1014
Miami Dade Fire Rescue Department, IAFF Local 1403
Fire Department-City of New York, IAFF Locals 94 & 854
Phoenix Fire Department, IAFF Local 493
Seattle Fire Department, IAFF Local 27

American Council on Exercise
Managing Editor: Daniel J. Green
Technical Editor: Cedric X. Bryant, Ph.D.
Director of Publications: Christine J. Ekeroth
Assistant Editor: Jennifer Schiffer
Cover design: Karen McGuire

Layout design: Jennifer Bokelmann
Front cover photo: Larry Steagall, *The West Sound Sun*, Bremerton, WA

Library of Congress Number: 2002109326
ISBN: 1-58518-708-9

Healthy Learning
P.O. Box 1828
Monterey, CA 93942
www.healthylearning.com

FOREWORD

Once again, the International Association of Fire Fighters and the International Association of Fire Chiefs have joined together in an unprecedented endeavor. We have set our sights on strengthening the foundation of the fire service – the fire fighter and EMS responder. We realize that meeting the challenges of tomorrow's fire service requires that we maintain the physical capability of uniformed personnel throughout their fire service career. To help us in this historic effort, we have gathered some of finest fire departments from the United States and Canada.

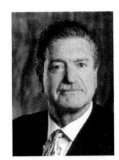

Harold A. Schaitberger
General President, IAFF

As promised, the Fire Service Joint Labor Management Wellness-Fitness Task Force has addressed improving fire fighter performance. The Wellness-Fitness Initiative was a critical move in improving fire fighter health, wellness, and fitness. The next step in the process was to hire physically capable candidates. In a bold proactive move, the Task Force, along with other technical experts, developed the comprehensive Candidate Physical Ability Testing (CPAT) program.

The IAFF and the IAFF/IAFC Task Force have agreed that to successfully implement the Wellness-Fitness Initiative and the CPAT, there must be fire fighters in each department who can take the lead. These individuals must have the ability to design and implement fitness programs, to improve the wellness and fitness of their department, and to assist with the physical training of recruits and members. This need for these department-level leaders led to the development of the Fire Service Peer Fitness Trainer (PFT) certification program.

After careful consideration of the major personal trainer certifying agencies, the American Council on Exercise (ACE) was chosen to collaborate in the development and implementation of the PFT certification program for fire fighters. ACE is a nonprofit organization dedicated to promoting the benefits of physical activity and protecting consumers against unsafe and ineffective fitness products and instruction. ACE is a standard-setting body for fitness professionals and the largest fitness certification and education provider in the world. As the nation's "workout watchdog," ACE also conducts university-based research and testing that targets fitness products and exercise programming trends.

The completion of this project could not have been possible without the professionalism and commitment of everyone involved. We recognize and applaud every member of this group for all the hard work they have done throughout the past two years. Our organizations will remain committed to developing programs to improve the quality of life of all fire fighters and emergency medical personnel.

ACKNOWLEDGEMENTS

The IAFF Department of Occupational Health and Safety would like to lend its appreciation and gratitude to those individuals who contributed their talent, knowledge, and expertise to the development and completion of the Fire Service Joint Labor Management Wellness-Fitness Initiative's Peer Fitness Trainer Certification Program and this *IAFF/IAFC/ACE Peer Fitness Trainer Manual.*

Foremost, to the leadership of the IAFF and the IAFC, especially to IAFF General President Harold A. Schaitberger and IAFC Presidents Michael Brown, John Buckman, and Randy Bruegman for their continued commitment on behalf of labor and management in meeting the challenge to design and implement an unprecedented program to change the face of the fire service with a certification program for Peer Fitness Trainers. Their foresight kept this labor/management effort on target as it addressed the health and safety of the fire service. Appreciation is offered to Vincent J. Bollon, IAFF General Secretary-Treasurer, for his supportive role throughout this endeavor and his desire for the continuation of this successful labor/management project. We also wish to recognize the valued efforts of Michael Crouse, IAFF Chief of Staff, for his direction and assistance in keeping this project on track.

Special acknowledgment is given to the IAFF Department of Health and Safety staff and consultants responsible for coordinating the Initiative process and manual. The Project Director, Raymond Wasdyke, Ed.D., guided the team in creating a valid, thorough, and effective certification program. Pat Morrison of the Fairfax County Fire Department and IAFF Local 2068 provided invaluable assistance as the chair of the PFT Advisory Committee. He was assisted by committee members Jill Craig, Austin Fire Department/IAFF Local 975; Anthony Boyce, Indianapolis Fire Department IAFF/Local 416; Derek Alkonis, Los Angeles County Fire Department/IAFF Local 1014; Scott Peltin, Phoenix Fire Department/IAFF Local 493; Olivia Templeton, Glendale Community College; Vicki Runnels, IAFC; and Ron McGraw, IAFF. Recognition is given to Ron Rogers, Ph.D., Psychometrician Consultant, Wasdyke Associates for his technical and communication skills; Andrea Kuettel for her technical review and editing skills; Dan Grove, Assistant to the General Secretary-Treasurer and Ricky Grant, Information Technology Assistant, for their knowledge and assistance with information technology; and Heather Knox, R.D., for her nutrition expertise.

The historic relationship that the IAFF established with the American Council on Exercise has made this joint certification project possible. We acknowledge ACE's Executive Director Ken Germano for his continued commitment and enthusiastic support in this endeavor. Also, we thank the following members of the ACE team: Cedric X. Bryant, Ph.D., Chief Exercise Physiologist/Vice President of Educational Services; Tony Ordas, Director of Certification; Daniel Green, Managing Editor; and Scott Goudeseune, Vice President of Sales & Business Development.

We are indebted to the following ten fire chiefs and IAFF local union presidents and their technical and operations staffs for the commitment of time and resources, and for their thoughtful direction and insight to the development of this certification effort. Each department and IAFF local union, regardless of the number of personnel committed to the project, participated equally to assure the Program's success.

- **Austin Fire Department:** Gary Warren, Fire Chief; Scott Toupin, President, IAFF Local 975; and Jill Craig, Fitness Coordinator.

- **Calgary Fire Department:** Wayne Morris, Fire Chief; David Wilcox, President, IAFF Local 255; and Fire Fighter Ian Crosby.

- **Charlotte Fire Department:** Luther Fincher, Fire Chief; Mike Spath, President, IAFF Local 660; and Glenn Jones, Physical Fitness Coordinator.

- **Fairfax County Fire and Rescue Department:** Edward Stinnette, Fire Chief; R. Michael Mohler, President, IAFF Local 2068; Pat Morrison, Lieutenant, Physical Fitness Coordinator; Nancy Kane, Physician Assistant; and Fire Fighter Stacie Lawton.

- **Indianapolis Fire Department:** Louis Dezelan, Fire Chief; Tom Hanify, President, IAFF Local 416; Julie Baade, Fitness Coordinator; Darrell Mendenhall, Exercise Physiologist; and Fire Fighters Anthony Boyce, Jason Kelly, and Roger Finchum.

- **Los Angeles County Fire Department:** Michael Freeman, Fire Chief; Richard Guererro, President, IAFF Local 1014; Derek Alkonis, Captain; George Cruz, Wellness-Fitness Coordinator; Bob Karwasky, Exercise Physiologist; and Fire Fighters Kevin Klar, Jan Chatelain, Brian Bennett, and Jeff Burke.

- **Miami Dade Fire Rescue Department:** Charles Phillips, Fire Chief; Dominick Barbera, President, IAFF Local 1403; Orlando Peña, Benefits Director, IAFF Local 1403; Cindy Sears, Assistant Director; and Fire Fighter Vesna McKenna.

- **New York City Fire Department:** Nicolas Scoppetta, Fire Commissioner; Stephen Cassidy, President, IAFF Local 94; Pete Gorman, President, IAFF Local 854; Kevin Malley, Lieutenant (Retired); and Michael Cacciola, Lieutenant, Fitness Program Director.

- **Phoenix Fire Department:** Alan Brunacini, Fire Chief; Billy Shields, President, IAFF Local 493; Scott Peltin, Division Chief; and Fire Fighters Andy Arredondo, Warren Bowden, and Lisa Jones.

- **Seattle Fire Department:** Gary Morris, Fire Chief; Paul Atwater, President, IAFF Local 27; and Kim Favorite, Physical Fitness Specialist.

We also express our gratitude to the United States Fire Administration for their financial support.

Richard M. Duffy
Assistant to the General President
Occupational Health, Safety and Medicine
International Association of Fire Fighters, AFL-CIO, CLC
1750 New York Avenue, NW
Washington, DC 20006

CONTENTS

INTRODUCTION

The goal of the *IAFF/IAFC/ACE Peer Fitness Trainer Reference Manual* was to take advantage of the expertise found at these two organizations to create a complement to the *ACE Personal Trainer Manual*. That manual, first published in 1991, has represented the fitness industry standard since it first appeared and is the core text used around the world as candidates prepare for the ACE personal trainer exam. But we knew that this book was not enough to prepare fire fighters for the role of Peer Fitness Trainer, as fire fighters have very specific fitness needs and an extreme work environment well beyond what the average exerciser will ever face. The manual you now hold in your hands provides the fire fighter–specific knowledge you will need to take recruits to the next level as you prepare them for the CPAT and for successful careers in the fire service.

Most of the chapters in this manual serve to complement chapters in the *ACE Personal Trainer Manual*. For example, Chapter Seven: Strength Training provides additional material on creating programs for fire fighters that goes beyond the scope of the strength training chapter in ACE's manual. The chapter offers a number of programming ideas that are specifically tailored to the needs and schedules of fire fighters, including various split routines and superset and compound set routines. Each type of workout is discussed in detail, as are the benefits to be gained from each.

Other chapters in this manual address topics not covered by the *ACE Personal Trainer Manual*. Chapters 1 and 6 are titled The Wellness-Fitness Initiative and IAFF/IAFC Candidate Physical Ability Test, respectively. These two chapters provide historical overviews of these programs and the rationale behind their development. Chapter 5, Fire Fighter Injury Prevention Guidelines, covers the many situations in which fire fighters become especially injury prone. This discussion includes everything from sleep deprivation and dehydration to unstable footing and working at one's maximum heart rate. Chapter 11, Fire Fighter–Specific Diseases, covers the many illness that are common in the fire service. While this information is not covered on the PFT exam, it is essential that PFTs, and indeed all fire fighters, be aware of the dangers of their work and take steps to ensure their own safety.

As a Peer Fitness Trainer, you are responsible for knowing and applying a significant amount of information. Your challenge is to use this information to safely and effectively train your fellow fire fighters and give them the results they need for a long and healthy career in the fire service. Remember, the primary goal of the IAFF and ACE in creating this certification program is to strengthen the fire service as a whole by strengthening it one fire fighter at a time.

Cedric X. Bryant, Ph.D.
Chief Exercise Physiologist/Vice President of Educational Services
American Council on Exercise

THE WELLNESS-FITNESS INITIATIVE

This chapter provides the PFT with a basic introduction to the IAFF/IAFC Joint Labor Management Wellness-Fitness Initiative (WFI). This chapter in no way replaces the actual WFI Manual, which must be followed in its entirety upon implementation of the program.

Historically, the fire service has paid more attention to its fire apparatus and equipment than the uniformed personnel who provide emergency services and use the equipment. Fire fighters and emergency medical services (EMS) personnel respond to emergency incidents that require extreme physical exertion. The high physical demands of the job often result in injuries and psychological stress, affecting the overall wellness of the fire fighting and emergency response system. In the past, the fire service has sought to improve wellness, fitness, and health by instituting fitness programs that rely solely on time-based performance tests. These tests were created to motivate fire fighters to improve their fitness by mandating that they meet a performance-based standard. These programs produced mediocre results and were often viewed as punitive by the personnel. In an effort to create a universally accepted program for improving health, wellness, and fitness within the North American fire service, the International Association of Fire Chiefs (IAFC) and the International Association of Fire Fighters (IAFF) joined efforts in 1996 to develop and implement the WFI.

The goal of the WFI is to improve the quality of life of all uniformed personnel. The WFI seeks to promote the value of investing in wellness resources over time to maintain fit, healthy, and capable fire fighters and EMS responders throughout their careers. Effective implementation of the full program should result in significant cost savings by reducing lost work time, workers' compensation, and disability for fire departments. In addition, participating departments will create an invaluable database to guide improvement in fire fighter health and safety.

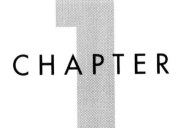

CHAPTER 1

Fire chiefs and IAFF local union presidents participating in the WFI have contributed to developing an overall wellness/fitness system with a holistic, positive, rehabilitating, and educational focus. All participants have committed themselves to moving beyond punitive, timed, task-based performance testing to progressive wellness improvement. Most importantly, all labor and management representatives jointly have committed themselves to implementing a wellness/fitness program that is specific to each fire fighter's needs and based on the recommendations in the WFI. Currently, hundreds of departments have adopted and implemented this program, building a stronger fire service by strengthening their fire fighters.

Table 1.1 The Ten Fire Departments from the United States and Canada that Participated in the Development of the Candidate Physical Ability Test

❑ Austin, Texas Fire Department

❑ Calgary, Alberta Fire Department

❑ Charlotte, North Carolina Fire Department

❑ Fairfax County, Virginia Fire and Rescue Department

❑ Indianapolis, Indiana Fire Department

❑ Los Angeles County, California Fire Department

❑ Miami Dade, Florida Fire Rescue Department

❑ City of New York, New York Fire Department

❑ Phoenix, Arizona Fire Department

❑ Seattle, Washington Fire Department

FIRE SERVICE JOINT LABOR MANAGEMENT WELLNESS-FITNESS INITIATIVE MISSION STATEMENT

Every fire department in cooperation with its local IAFF affiliate must develop an overall wellness/fitness system to maintain the physical and mental capabilities of uniformed personnel. While such a program may be mandatory, agreement to initiate it must be mutual between the administration and its members represented by the local union. Any program of physical fitness must be positive and not punitive in design; require mandatory participation by all uniformed personnel once implemented; make allowances for age, gender, and position in the department; allow for on-duty participation utilizing facilities and equipment provided or arranged by the department; provide for rehabilitation and remedial support for those in need; contain training and education components; and, be reasonable and equitable to all participants. The program should be long-term, and, where possible, be made available to retirees. All wellness/fitness programs must include the following key elements:

➤ Behavioral, medical, and fitness evaluations that are kept confidential and secure

➤ Physical fitness and wellness programs that are educational and rehabilitative, and not punitive

➤ Performance testing that promotes progressive wellness improvement

➤ Labor and management committed to a positive individualized fitness/wellness program

The WFI focuses on five main areas: medical evaluation, fitness testing and exercise, rehabilitation, behavioral health promotion, and data collection. This chapter provides only a brief synopsis of the information contained in the WFI. It is strongly recommended that the complete document be ordered through the IAFF or IAFC and read in its entirety.

MEDICAL

The medical exam outlined in the WFI is different from a typical annual "check-up." The information collected in this exam is specific to fire department uniformed personnel and is designed to help identify health problems affecting the individual, his or her department, and the professional fire service. Medical, fitness, and injury data are gathered annually to track the history and health status of fire fighters and EMS providers as a group.

The medical exam presented in the WFI is designed to accomplish the following:

✓ Determine, through the fire department physician, whether an individual is physically and mentally able to perform essential job duties without undue risk of harm to self or others

✓ Monitor the effects of exposure to specific biological, physical, or chemical agents

✓ Detect changes in an individual's health that may be related to harmful working conditions

✓ Detect any patterns of disease in the workforce that might indicate underlying work-related problems

✓ Provide the worker with information about his or her occupational hazards and current health

✓ Provide a cost-effective investment in disease prevention and health promotion in fire fighters

✓ Comply with federal, state, provincial, and local requirements

FITNESS

Throughout the history of the fire service, the proper implementation of fitness programs in fire departments has been extensively debated. Research has shown the need for high levels of aerobic fitness, muscular endurance, and muscular strength to perform fire fighting job tasks safely and effectively (Kenney & Landy, 1998; Jackson, 1994; Shepard, 1991). Physical fitness is critical to maintaining the wellness of our uniformed personnel and therefore must be incorporated into the overall fire service philosophy and culture.

Assessment of uniformed personnel current fitness levels is an important part of developing an individualized fitness program. However, assessment is not in itself a fitness program. An effective physical fitness program has several required components, including the following:

- ✓ Fitness evaluations

- ✓ Qualified PFTs and exercise specialists

- ✓ On-duty workout time

- ✓ Availability of safe workout equipment and facilities

- ✓ Incorporation of fitness into fire department philosophy and culture through education and awareness

- ✓ Individualized fitness programming

The PFTs will play a critical role in determining the success of any wellness/fitness program. An integrated multi-level approach in which an exercise professional trains and oversees multiple PFTs is recommended. For PFTs to provide accurate and safe information they should complete a certified comprehensive course (and obtain professional certification) that provides broad scientific knowledge of exercise, and understanding of proper exercise technique.

Certification improves the credibility and safety of departmental fitness programs, but is only the first step. In order for PFTs to remain competent and improve the quality of their wellness/fitness programs, continuing education is essential. This may include taking college exercise science courses, attending workshops and symposiums, and reading professional journals.

Qualified Peer Fitness Trainers can contribute to fire departments in many ways, including the following:

- Educating company officers about the benefits of wellness and fitness for their crew members

- Educating new hires regarding the importance of wellness and fitness throughout their fire service careers

- Educating fire department members about the benefits of wellness and fitness

- Performing yearly fitness assessments of incumbents

- Evaluating and selecting fitness equipment

- Designing and supporting personalized fitness programs for fire department members
- Teaching Fire FitKids classes as part of the fire department's and IAFF's community outreach
- Participating in recruiting and mentoring programs for the fire department
- Designing and teaching preparatory classes for potential fire department recruits

FITNESS EVALUATIONS

The WFI requires all uniformed personnel to participate in mandatory annual, non-punitive, and confidential fitness assessments following medical clearance. After each fitness assessment is completed, the PFT should provide feedback to the individual and the department's physician regarding the individual's physical capacity to perform their job. This personalized feedback includes the individual's current level of fitness, level of improvement since past assessments, a realistic evaluation of his or her physical capacity to safely perform assigned jobs, and a suggested exercise program. In addition, some of the data collected is entered into a confidential database to be used for future fire service research.

All uniformed personnel must understand that the goal of these evaluations is solely for personal fitness improvement. No standards are mandated by the WFI for any of these areas. Each uniformed person is expected to improve with an assessment and a personalized exercise program. The following is a detailed explanation of the assessment in each of four specific areas.

AEROBIC CAPACITY

According to each IAFF Death and Injury Survey since 1981, the leading occupation-related diseases causing premature departures from the fire service were heart disease and lung disease. Aerobic fitness may improve individual resistance to these two categories of disease.

Aerobic fitness is fundamental to the health, safety, and performance of all uniformed personnel. A program of regular aerobic exercise can help improve cardiovascular fitness and maintain normal body composition, blood pressure, cholesterol, and blood sugar levels. Research has demonstrated that inactive persons have a 90% higher risk of heart attack than physically active persons.

Numerous studies have demonstrated the necessity of maintaining a high level of aerobic capacity for fire service duties (Kenney & Landy, 1998; Jackson, 1994; Shepard, 1991). Measurements of heart rate response taken during normal fire fighting tasks have been shown to be at, or near, maximal levels. In addition, the oxygen consumption rates associated with the performance of live fire, rescue, and suppression tasks fall within the range of 9 to 12 METs (or 31.5 to 42.0 ml/kg/min). The cardiovascular, respiratory, and thermoregulatory strain resulting from the performance of work at this high level of intensity is profound. Thus, optimal aerobic capacity is essential for the safety of the member and the performance of his or her job.

Aerobic capacity can be evaluated in many ways. The most accurate measurement will be the one that most closely simulates the fire fighter's job requirements. The WFI requires the use of either treadmill or stairmill.

Measurements of aerobic capacity are done at sub-maximal or maximal levels. Sub-maximal aerobic capacity tests, when properly validated, have been shown to accurately estimate the individual's maximal aerobic capacity ($\dot{V}O_2$max). These tests are less expensive and easier to administer than maximal tests, and can be performed in a fitness center setting by a qualified fitness professional. See page 68 for these protocols.

For those departments electing to use maximal aerobic capacity tests, only trained and certified personnel under the direct supervision of the fire department physician can administer such tests. Testing must be conducted in a medical care setting with EKG monitoring and resuscitation equipment available.

Aerobic Capacity Evaluations

The Wellness-Fitness Initiative provides two protocols to estimate a fire fighter's maximal aerobic capacity through a submaximal effort: the Gerkin sub-maximal treadmill protocol and the Fire Department of New York (FDNY) sub-maximal stairmill protocol. Both protocols estimate a fire fighter's maximal aerobic capacity (expressed as $\dot{V}O_2$max) using the calculations provided in the respective sections.

Either of these two protocols can be used by fire departments adopting the Wellness-Fitness Initiative. The chosen protocol must be used consistently for all uniformed personnel within that department, and the protocol must be recorded for data entry. Results of aerobic capacity over time can be compared only if the same protocol is used. If a fire department changes protocols, a new baseline $\dot{V}O_2$max must be established for each individual. All aerobic capacity evaluation results must be recorded in milligrams of oxygen per kilograms of body weight per minute (ml/kg/min).

Muscular Strength

Strength is defined as the maximal force that a specific muscle or muscle group can generate. The demands of fire fighting require above-average strength. Several studies and job analyses have shown that the weight of equipment used by a single fire fighter on the job is in excess of 100 pounds. (Gledhill & Jamnik, 1992; Lemon & Hermiston, 1977; Goldstein et al., 1996). Reduced muscular strength can contribute to the high incidence of sprains, strains, and back injuries among fire fighters.

Strength measurements are specific to the joint and range of motion being measured. Since uniformed personnel require strength in multiple areas for successful and safe job performance, multiple areas should be measured. Strength measurement requires an individual to execute a maximal muscular contraction, which can be inherently unsafe. To measure strength accurately with the highest degree of safety, evaluators must emphasize proper technique.

For safety and data collection purposes, strength measurements are assessed by the grip dynamometer, leg dynamometer, and arm dynamometer evaluations. These are all safe, valid, and reliable methods to measure muscular strength.

Grip strength has been shown to be a key factor in many essential emergency service tasks, including the following:

- Lifting and carrying equipment
- Removing victims
- Holding and operating hose lines
- Raising extension ladders
- Patient transport

Grip strength is measured using a handgrip dynamometer. See page 76 for the handgrip protocol.

Leg strength is required for many essential emergency service tasks, including:

- Lifting and carrying equipment
- Forcing entry
- Climbing and negotiating ladders and stairs
- Pulling and operating hose lines
- Patient transport

Leg strength is measured using a leg dynamometer. See page 77 for the leg strength protocol.

Arm flexion strength is key for performing many standard and essential fire and emergency tasks, including:

- Stabilizing, lifting, and carrying tools and equipment
- Operating handlines
- Patient transport

Arm strength is measured using the same dynamometer used for the leg press evaluation. See page 78 for the arm strength protocol.

Muscular Endurance

Muscular endurance is the ability of a muscle group to perform repeated contractions. Several studies and job analyses have shown a strong association between muscular endurance and the essential job tasks of fire fighting (Kenney & Landy, 1998; Jackson, 1994; Shepard, 1991). Low levels of muscular endurance contribute to many preventable fire service injuries. For example, abdominal muscle endurance is necessary to stabilize the torso and support the lower back during exertion. Weak abdominal muscles may contribute to low-back pain and low-back injury. The curl-up test is used to measure muscular endurance of the abdominal muscles. See page 80 for this protocol.

The push-up test will be used to measure upper-body muscular endurance. The push-up test is a measure of the muscular endurance of the pectorals and the triceps. See page 79 for this protocol.

Flexibility

Flexibility is the functional measure of the range of motion of a joint. It is dependent on the pliability of the surrounding tissues (i.e., muscles, tendons, and ligaments). Although the effect of increasing flexibility on performance is controversial, it is widely accepted that a lack of flexibility may be a major contributor to injuries. Joint and limb restrictions can influence essential dynamic movements, balance, coordination, and muscular work efficiency.

According to each IAFF Death and Injury Survey since 1981, the leading type of line-of-duty injury within the professional fire service is sprains and strains. In addition, back injury is the most prevalent line-of-duty injury leading to premature departure from the fire service. Low levels of flexibility very likely contributed to these statistics. When a joint lacks flexibility, it is unable to move safely through a normal range of motion. Once this occurs, other surrounding joints must compensate to perform essential tasks. This biomechanical compromise can lead to injuries.

The Miami Dade County Fire Rescue Department recently reported that 55% of their members reported current low-back pain. In addition, 86% of members reported a past medical history of low-back pain. It is critical, therefore, that assessment procedures do not exacerbate these symptoms or cause further injury.

For the purposes of the WFI, trunk flexion is evaluated by the sit-and-reach test. This test is commonly used to assess trunk function. The test is administered according to the sit and reach test protocol method outlined on page 81.

Data Collection of Fitness Evaluation

The goal of data collection described in this Initiative is to collect long-term information on the health and fitness of fire service personnel to assess the medical and fitness history of a large group of fire fighters and determine the impact of the program. The data collected from the fitness assessments will identify the following:

- Aerobic capacity, flexibility, muscular strength, and muscular endurance of all uniformed personnel

- Changes in fitness levels of personnel over their careers

- Effectiveness of the medical and fitness program in improving individual physical fitness levels

- Muscular weaknesses and imbalances in individuals, which may contribute to future injuries if left uncorrected

- Possible risk factors for back injury

- Possible factors associated with musculoskeletal injuries in fire service personnel

The complete data collection protocol for the WFI Database is found in Chapter 6 of the WFI Manual. The following is an overview of the fitness component data points.

FITNESS DATA QUESTIONS	
In an average week during the past month, how often did you walk a mile or more at a time without stopping?	
In an average week during the past month, how often did you engage in aerobic exercise for 20 minutes or more without stopping?	
In an average week during the past month, how often did you lift weights?	
Compared with yourself one year ago, would you say that you are more active now, less active now, or about the same?	
Record Fitness Test Scores: **Aerobic Capacity**	
Test type (treadmill or stairmill)	
Capacity (ml O_2/minute)	
Capacity (ml O_2/kg of body weight/minute)	
Muscular Strength	
Hand Dynamometer (kg)	
Leg Dynamometer (kg)	
Arm Dynamometer (kg)	
Muscular Endurance	
Push-Up (# performed in two minutes; 80 max)	
Curl-Up (# performed in three minutes; 60 max)	
Flexibility	
Modified Sit and Reach (inches)	

Self-Assessment

The WFI self-assessment gives fire fighters valuable feedback on individual fitness levels, ability to recover from exertion, and overall physical capacity. It is an evaluation that fire fighters can safely perform without assistance to provide feedback on level of fitness, level of improvement, and physical capacity for exercise. The exercises, weights, repetitions, and aerobic equipment chosen for use in a self-assessment should reflect the actual job demands. The fitness circuit protocol, shown on page 85, is an innovative application of a self-assessment related to the job of fire fighting.

A self-assessment can be performed at the workout location with minimal equipment. The information collected from the assessment can be compared to previous and future assessments. For example, if an individual's heart rate at one minute exceeds 90% of the estimated maximum, that individual may lack the reserve necessary to perform safely on the fireground. Similarly, if an individual is unable to complete the required repetitions for a particular exercise, that individual may be unable to sufficiently complete the essential task that the exercise simulates. This information should be used to motivate fire fighters to improve any deficiencies noted during the evaluation.

INDIVIDUAL EXERCISE PROGRAMMING

Individual exercise programs are essential to the WFI. Each personalized progressive plan accounts for the individual's current level of fitness, job duties, time restrictions, physical capabilities, nutritional status, and self-improvement efforts. Mass exercise programs, not tailored for the individual, are destined to fail.

Although personalized fitness programs are more time-consuming and costly, the benefits cannot be overstated. The customer service element of exercise programming is critical. The fitness assessment previously described is only the first step in educating fire fighters about their levels of fitness and guiding them in establishing specific personal goals. Assessment must be followed by one-on-one consultations in which individuals can address concerns and learn about recommended exercises and equipment.

Personalized exercise programs should consider the following individual characteristics:

- Age
- Weight
- Motivation level
- Goals
- Current aerobic capacity
- Current fitness level
- Current and previous injuries and disabilities
- History and experience of working out

- Physical work requirements

- Muscle imbalances

- Personal lifestyle

- Time constraints

- Equipment available

- Preferred exercises and activities

- Sociological motivation (individual or group)

In addition, the program should focus on making acceptable lifestyle changes, including changes in nutrition, time management, and priorities. Similarly, the program must be balanced to include each fitness area:

- ✓ Cardiovascular training

- ✓ Flexibility training

- ✓ Muscular strength training

- ✓ Muscular endurance training

In some cases, job-orientated task-performance exercise programs may be appropriate. All programs should be progressive in nature and should always err on the side of slower progression, lighter weights, and undertraining instead of overtraining. Job-specific allowances must be considered, allowing for sleep deprivation, high stress shifts, and excessive workload (e.g., working fires, long incidents, heavy rescues, or high number of calls). Fire fighters have been referred to as professional athletes when in fact they are occupational athletes. The term occupational athletes accurately reflects the numerous uncontrollable variables that are part of the job and must be considered when designing individual exercise programs.

INJURY/MEDICAL/FITNESS REHABILITATION

Every year, statistics show that fire fighting is one of the most dangerous occupations in the world. In some departments, medical disability from occupational injuries and illnesses accounts for over 50% of the retirements. According to the 1999 IAFF Death and Injury Survey, low-back injuries and other sprains and strains accounted for 57.2% of total injuries. Fire fighter injuries caused 2,872 lost work hours per 100 workers.

When compared to data compiled for private industry by the United States Bureau of Labor Statistics, the IAFF Death and Injury Survey indicates that the frequency of fire fighter job-related injury is 8.6 times that of workers in private industry. If this trend continues, at least one out of every three fire fighters will be injured annually. The fire department must take the lead in ensuring that fire fighters are properly rehabilitated prior to returning to full duty. When assessing the functional capacities of fire fighters after significant injuries or illnesses, physicians and therapists familiar with fire fighting job requirements should make informed decisions. In short, the fire department must control the process and provide the necessary input to drive this process; and, labor must support the rehabilitation process from beginning to end.

Any fire fighter on extended leave from normal duties for a continuous period of six months or more must undergo medical and fitness evaluations before returning to full duty. Extended leave status includes alternate assignment, leave of absence, and leave due to illness, injury, pregnancy, or other qualifying situation. This practice will help identify loss of conditioning, which may put fire fighters at risk for future injuries.

INJURY PREVENTION

A proactive injury prevention program must be implemented to reduce risks in the fire service and improve personnel resistance to injuries. Program components include the following:

- ✓ A comprehensive and effective wellness program

- ✓ A physical fitness program

- ✓ A strong commitment to safety from both labor and management

- ✓ A designated safety officer

- ✓ An ergonomic analysis of all aspects of the job to determine where redesign of the work environment is needed

- ✓ An educational component that begins in the fire academy and continues throughout the entire career

- ✓ A recognition system for personnel who preach and practice safety

BEHAVIORAL HEALTH

A wellness program is not complete without addressing the behavioral health of those involved. The behavioral health of uniformed personnel is essential to their physical health and well-being. With the recent development of Employee Assistance Programs and Critical Incident Stress Debriefing Programs, behavioral health issues within the fire service are receiving more attention. The behavioral health component of WFI provides important tools to assist all uniformed personnel in achieving total wellness. The services available through behavioral health must ensure confidentiality and privacy for uniformed personnel both in writing and in practice.

To maintain a high level of job performance, uniformed personnel must be able to cope effectively with the emotional, physical, and mental stresses of work and personal life. If the ability to cope becomes compromised, these stresses may negatively impact a fire fighter's mental and emotional health. Co-worker injury or death, financial distress, marital and family problems, alcoholism, drug addiction, and occupational stress may be affecting the individual both on and off the job.

NUTRITION

The demands of the job on fire fighters are great. The fuel necessary to meet these demands is found in the individual's diet. Proper nutrition is a must, as it enhances the performance and quality of life of all fire fighters.

Aside from the limits imposed by heredity and the physical performance improvements associated with training, no factor plays a bigger role in exercise performance than nutrition. The benefits of a well balanced diet include the following:

❑ Feeling better day to day

❑ More energy to exercise harder and for longer durations

❑ Quicker recovery after workouts and after difficult incidents

❑ Improved resistance to diseases

Obesity increases an individual's risk for injury, reduces performance, and adversely affects the ability to dissipate heat while working. A well balanced diet, combined with a consistent exercise program, is the most reliable method to reduce body fat.

A dietitian is a valuable asset to any wellness program. The field of nutrition is plagued with fads and misinformation. Members, company officers, supervisors, and PFTs can benefit from the expertise that a dietitian can offer. These experts can be retained by contract, as volunteers, or through internships or similar arrangements. Some of the benefits of a dietitian include the following:

❑ Developing weight management programs

❑ Analyzing individual diets

❑ Customizing diet programs (e.g., pregnancy, weight gain, or illness)

❑ Educating Peer Fitness Trainers, company officers, members, and recruits

❑ Developing specialized meals for nutritional replenishment after incidents

❑ Meeting with counselors to assist obese members seeking behavioral modification intervention

BODY COMPOSITION

Body composition is a component of overall physical fitness. The ratio of fat to lean body mass has significant implications in both general health and physical performance. Body composition can be estimated through skinfold measures (by using calipers); hydrostatic, or underwater, weighing; bioelectrical impedance; height/weight ratio (body mass index); and circumference measurements.

The WFI does not include a protocol for estimating body composition and will not collect body composition data, for several reasons. Each of the body composition testing methods has inherent advantages and disadvantages. Some are more vulnerable than others to technician error. Some methods require that the individual be assessed at the same degree of hydration each time to be accurate. Some are uncomfortable, or require expensive equipment and a great deal of time to perform, or require that the participant expose specific anatomical sites. And still these "indirect measures" are, at best, approximations.

This is not to say that estimating body composition should be discouraged. Each department should take into consideration several factors before performing body composition testing: the experience of the personnel conducting the assessment, the means available to the department, the time allotted for the assessment, the accuracy of the method, and the cost.

DATA COLLECTION

The data component of the WFI includes the storage and analysis of detailed case information related to medical conditions (exam/laboratory data), fitness, rehabilitation, and behavioral health. The data collection system must include uniform, consistent, and efficient collection of information from participating fire departments and data compilation in an international database for analysis. To accomplish this, participating fire departments must utilize key components: a local fire department information system, an established data dictionary, and specific file transfer specifications. The WFI data is uploaded into the International Wellness-Fitness Database.

All health-related data collected by the International Wellness-Fitness Database is confidential. Individual identities are not submitted by the fire department to the database for any job history, annual medical and fitness evaluation, or injury data. The goal of data collection described in the WFI is to provide information that will assess the medical and fitness history of the fire fighter and determine the impact of the Wellness-Fitness program.

REFERENCES

Gledhill, N. & Jamnik, V.K. (1992). Characterization of the physical demands of fire fighting, *Canadian Journal of Sport Science*, 17, 3, 207–213.

Goldstein, A. et al. (1996). *Exercise performance of New York City fire fighters wearing various protective uniform ensembles.* Commissioner's Report.

Kenney, W.L. & Landy, F.J. (1998). Fitness testing for fire fighters. *ACSM's Health and Fitness Journal*, 2, 12–17.

Lemon, P.W.R. & Hermiston, R.T. (1977). The energy cost of fire fighting. *Journal of Occupational Medicine*, 19, 337–340.

Jackson, A.S. (1994). Pre-employment physical education. *Exercise and Sport Sciences Reviews*, 22, 53–90.

Shepard, R.J. (1991). Occupational demand and human rights: Public safety officers and cardiorespiratory fitness. *Sports Medicine*, 12, 94–109.

PROFESSIONAL
RESPONSIBILITY

The role of a PFT is a privileged one, and you have a personal obligation to act in a professional and responsible manner. Many PFTs also have credentials in other disciplines (e.g., EMT or paramedic) and are obligated to know and follow the ethical standards of their professional boards.

KNOW THE SCOPE OF PRACTICE

PFTs have an obligation to be knowledgeable in a wide variety of areas including exercise science, anatomy, physiology, assessment, exercise programming, behavior change, and basic nutrition. However, PFTs are not qualified to diagnose injuries or provide treatment. PFTs are not equipped to deal with psychological problems or psychiatric illnesses such as depression or eating disorders (e.g., anorexia nervosa and bulimia). While general nutritional recommendations related to decreasing fat consumption and eating more complex carbohydrates are common, prescribing a specific diet with food, vitamins, and calorie consumption may be regulated by the state and require the license of a registered dietitian or nutritionist. PFTs must know the scope and limits of their practice and refrain from advising in subject areas for which they have no formal training or lack the proper credentials.

The scope of practice for a certified PFT is summarized as follows:

Individual Assessment

- Provide a strong rationale for a fitness program
- Gather relevant information from participants
- Identify health risk factors
- Conduct fitness assessments
- Recognize warning signs and/or symptoms
- Establish follow-up criteria

CHAPTER

Program Design

- Integrate assessment results and individual goals
- Design a comprehensive exercise program
- Individualize the training program

Program Implementation

- Encourage adherence
- Employ multi-sensory learning modalities
- Recognize warning signs
- Teach correct biomechanical techniques

Program Administration

- Evaluate/inspect exercise equipment
- Document essential findings
- Maintain integrity and credibility
- Evaluate program effectiveness
- Promote peer trainer services

It is not uncommon for a fire fighter to ask a PFT for information that lies beyond his or her scope of practice. Some examples of services that a PFT should NOT offer are listed below and discussed in Table 2.1.

- ❏ Diagnose an injury
- ❏ Prescribe a course of treatment for an injury or illness
- ❏ Advise a fire fighter to take specific dietary supplements or performance enhancement agents
- ❏ Provide a specific nutritional/dietary program
- ❏ Counsel a fire fighter regarding a behavioral disorder

Table 2.1 IDEA Personal Fitness Trainers' Scope of Practice and Appropriate Terminology

Fitness Professionals DO NOT:	Fitness Professionals DO:
diagnose	• receive exercise, health, or nutrition guidelines from a physician, physical therapist, registered dietitian, etc. • follow national consensus guidelines for exercise programming for medical disorders • screen for exercise limitations • identify potential risk factors through screening • refer clients to an appropriate allied health professional or medical practitioner
prescribe	• design exercise programs • refer clients to an appropriate allied health professional or medical practitioner for an exercise prescription
prescribe diets or recommend specific supplements	• provide general information on healthy eating, according to the USDA Food Guide Pyramid • refer clients to a dietitian or nutritionist for a specific diet plan
treat injury or disease	• refer clients to an appropriate allied health professional or medical practitioner for treatment • use exercise to help improve overall health • help clients follow physician or therapist advice
monitor progress for medically-referred fire fighters	• document progress • report progress to an appropriate allied health professional or medical practitioner • follow physician, therapist, or dietitian recommendations
rehabilitate	• design an exercise program once a client has been released from rehabilitation
counsel	• coach • provide general information • refer clients to a qualified counselor or therapist
work with patients	• work with clients

Source: IDEA Health & Fitness Association's Opinion Statement: Benefits of a Working Relationship Between Medical and Allied Health Practitioners and Personal Fitness Trainers

ESTABLISH REFERRAL NETWORKS

A skilled trainer will establish a network of professionals in related disciplines for fire fighter referral, such as physicians for general medical care and exercise clearance, orthopedic specialists for joint and back difficulties, registered dieticians for specific nutritional counseling, and psychologists or other mental health professionals for psychological counseling when warranted. By working directly with known trustworthy referral sources, fire fighters are more likely to receive continuity of care. Additionally, these professionals can serve as invaluable referral sources to the PFT.

PROTECT FIRE FIGHTER CONFIDENTIALITY

PFTs have both legal and moral obligations to protect the confidentiality of all information that fire fighters provide them. PFTs are obligated to keep private the names, records, and information related to all fire fighters. More importantly, all fire fighters have a right to expect that what they discuss will be kept private except where a legal statute dictates otherwise or when they have provided explicit written consent authorizing the PFT to disclose information to another specified individual.

Most breaches of confidentiality are not deliberate acts. Rather, they occur inadvertently. For example, Michael works as a PFT in a city fire department. When at the fire station, he uses a study room as an office, filing his fire fighter records in a folder marked with his name. He pulls them before his appointments, and then returns them to this folder in the file cabinet at the station. This is a potential breach of confidentiality. The names of all his fire fighters, their assessments, and their records could be seen by any other fire fighter or any officer with access to the study room. Fire fighter names and assessment data are privileged information and must be kept confidential. Neither the file cabinet nor the study room are kept locked, so they could be viewed by any other fire fighter during any other shift. Files must be kept in a locked cabinet with restricted access, or in a computer file secured by a password.

KEEP ACCURATE RECORDS

Many professionals have specific mandates for appropriate record keeping. PFTs must keep appropriate records of each meeting with a fire fighter and of meetings that are scheduled but cancelled for any reason. It is good practice to document carefully the initial assessment and goals, planned interventions, medical history, and exercise clearance. Any contact with relevant healthcare providers (e.g., physician, physical therapist) should also be recorded. All sessions must be documented briefly with date, length of session, topics discussed, goals established, and activity completed. PFTs may wish to keep fire fighters' exercise records on file as well.

PREFERENCES AND BIASES

Health and fitness professionals, like everyone, have their own personal preferences and biases. Age, gender, ethnic, and personal differences abound in an increasingly diverse fire service. Sensitivity to individual differences, as well as familiarity with social practices and philosophies of other cultures, is highly recommended. What distinguishes an effective Peer Fitness Trainer from an ineffective one is the degree to which these biases influence and interfere with the best interest of the fire fighter. For example, a possibly detrimental personal bias is the passionate belief that traditional aerobic classes are the key to total fitness. While this type of exercise will benefit many fire fighters, it may be inappropriate for others, such as those individuals with a history of knee, back, or foot problems. Also, current research suggests that lifestyle activity (e.g., walking, gardening, short bouts of activity throughout the day) also may be effective in managing weight and improving risk factor profiles. The trainer who rigidly recommends the same exercise for all fire fighters is providing a disservice to the fire service. PFTs are obligated to look for the best fit between activity and individual preference and lifestyle.

STAY CURRENT

PFTs reflect a blending of many disciplines. To become certified, a broad area of knowledge from many disciplines is required. However, certification as a Peer Fitness Trainer is just the beginning. Ongoing professional development and education is required to maintain certification status and to keep in touch with accurate, up-to-date information. With hormones, medications, and genetic therapy for weight control in the news nearly every week, PFTs must stay current through professional training, workshops, reading, and conferences.

For more information on obtaining required continuing education credit, please refer to the IAFF Department of Health and Safety.

THE STANDARD OF CARE

Individuals engaged in the delivery of public services have a duty to render that service in accordance with the established "standards of care." Deviation from those standards can be legally challenged if substandard care causes harm and damage to a client.

In the fitness and wellness industry, a variety of written standards of accountability exist that establish benchmarks of expected behavior for those providing the service. Standards of accountability for the fitness industry are provided by the American Heart Association (AHA), the American College of Sports Medicine (ACSM), the American Council on Exercise (ACE), the American Physical Therapy Association (APTA), the American Association of Cardiovascular & Pulmonary Rehabilitation (AACVPR), the American Medical Association (AMA), the American College of Cardiology (ACC), the International Health, Racquet, and Sportsclub Association (IHRSA), the National Strength and Conditioning Association (NSCA), and the Young Men's Christian Association (YMCA). These, and other organizations, provide written standards of expected behavior that can be used in legal proceedings to establish expected parameters of care. The standards provide information and direction in the areas of fire fighter screening, assessment, and recommendations for activity, supervision, emergency response, and documentation. In this regard, PFTs have an obligation, prior to recommending activity, to obtain sufficient information from a fire fighter to determine if that fire fighter can, upon assessment of that information, safely carry on the recommended activity. ACSM standards specify that a health history questionnaire or a PAR-Q–type form must be obtained and analyzed before activity is recommended to a consumer by a wellness/fitness professional. If such a screening device indicates that medical clearance is necessary before a fire fighter begins activity, then such a clearance must be obtained prior to recommending the activity. Should the fire fighter neglect or refuse to obtain clearance, the ACSM standards specify that no activity recommendations be provided. PFTs may be liable for deviations from such written standards if a fire fighter is injured as a result. Consequently, it is important for the PFT to comply with the published standards, not only for screening and assessing fire fighters, but also for recommending and supervising activity, and providing emergency response if needed.

PFTs should be aware of the fact that the standards of care for service delivery to fire fighters are constantly changing. As new scientific or professional developments unfold in this practice area, the standards of care will inevitably change. As a consequence, PFTs will need to stay abreast of the developments in this field in the same manner as they would in the field of emergency response.

One of the most practical ways to stay on top of professionally important changes to the standard of care is to participate in continuing education and similar programs. In addition, PFTs clearly have an obligation to keep current with professional publications and resources that might have an impact on their ability to provide better service to fire fighters. Trainers who neglect these continuing education and self-development requirements run the risk of providing services that do not meet current standards of care and losing certification status.

STATE REGULATION OF HEALTH CARE

Professional delivery of services to consumers is frequently subjected to local, state, and/or federal regulation. Such regulations take many forms and cover a host of activities, from door-to-door sales to the practice of medicine and other healthcare services. State laws generally regulate healthcare professionals and the delivery of healthcare services, although there may be relevant federal and local regulations as well.

State law in virtually all jurisdictions governs the practice of medicine, nursing, dentistry, chiropractic medicine, and physical therapy. Athletic training, various other therapies, and the practice of dieticians/nutritionists are also regulated in many jurisdictions. Some emerging professional services, such as clinical exercise physiology, are now subject to state regulation through the enactment of licensing statutes.

State licensing statutes for various service providers differ from state to state. Moreover, the roles, responsibilities, and obligations specified by law may be overlapping or ill defined. As a result, a sometimes-confusing patchwork of state laws is imposed upon healthcare providers and allied health professionals. Despite these overlapping or poorly defined boundaries, individuals must ensure that they are entitled to provide specified services with or without licensure, registration, or certification by that jurisdiction. To make that determination, individuals involved in personal training and lifestyle and weight management consulting must determine what they can and cannot do under particular state laws and regulations in the jurisdiction in which they deliver services. It may be necessary to consult with an attorney and/or state-regulating agency regarding local statutes. If the service area is subject to state control, PFTs must comply with the requirements before delivering that service. This may include passing a certification exam, or becoming licensed or registered. The PFT must know the scope of practice, and obtain the required credentials before delivering regulated services. Otherwise, the PFT risks legal liability.

PROMOTING THE PEER FITNESS TRAINER PROGRAM

The success of the PFT program in a fire department depends heavily on how well the program is publicized and promoted. There are several initiatives that PFTs can undertake to ensure that all fire fighters are aware of the program. Increasing fire fighter awareness enhances their likelihood of involvement, either as PFTs themselves or as recipients of the PFT services.

The PFT is responsible for introducing the newly launched PFT program. This can best be accomplished by visiting fire stations to give presentations or, if this is impractical, by giving presentations via teleconference heard in all stations. Producing a short introductory video to be distributed to each fire station is another cost-effective way of outlining the key elements of the program.

The introduction should be very positive, as some fire fighters may view the program as a way to showcase their weaknesses. Place emphasis on the program's goals of achieving improved overall wellness and fitness and strengthening peer relationships within the department.

The PFT may also consider launching a department newsletter to further promote the program. Such a newsletter may feature articles on wellness and fitness, fitness myths and facts, nutrition, and "success stories" if participants are willing to share them.

Perhaps the best advertisements for the PFT program are the PFTs themselves. A PFT's professionalism, integrity, knowledge, and interpersonal skills benefit not only the fire fighter, but also the overall program. The merits of the PFT and the program will spread by word of mouth encouraging more people to become involved.

Even with the most dedicated PFTs and most motivated fire fighters, support from the fire chief and fire fighters' union is another integral component of the PFT program's success. Obviously, improved wellness and fitness are linked to fire fighter health and safety, so all interests are best served by allocating necessary funds to establish such a program. An added, immeasurable facet of the program is enhanced peer relationships, resulting from the PFT and fire fighter working together toward a common goal not directly relating to the fireground.

Ideally, the PFT will have other resources and creative ideas about how to showcase the

PFT program, why it has been implemented, and how it works and how a fire fighter can benefit from it. Slightly different approaches to marketing the program can be used to recruit both new fire fighters and new PFT prospects, resulting in continued growth of the program.

Professional Resources

American College of Sports Medicine (ACSM)
P.O. Box 1440
Indianapolis, IN 46206-1440
317-637-9200 Fax 317-634-7817
www.acsm.org

With more than 18,000 members worldwide, the American College of Sports Medicine promotes and integrates scientific research, education, and practical applications of sports medicine and exercise science to maintain and enhance physical performance, fitness, health, and quality of life.

American Council on Exercise (ACE)
4851 Paramount Drive
San Diego, CA 92123
1-800-825-3636
www.acefitness.org

The American Council on Exercise (ACE) is a non-profit consumer protection organization that helps people enjoy safe and effective exercise. ACE sets the standard for certifying fitness professionals and informs the public about the safety and effectiveness of fitness products and programs. ACE offers certification for personal trainers, group fitness instructors, lifestyle and weight management consultants, and clinical exercise specialists. There are currently more than 40,000 active ACE-certified Professionals in the United States and 77 other countries.

American Heart Association (AHA)
7272 Greenville Ave.
Dallas, TX 75231
214-706-1179 Fax 1-800-242-8721
www.americanheart.org

The American Heart Association is a voluntary health agency whose primary mission is the reduction of death and disability due to heart disease and stroke. By providing a variety of worksite, schoolsite, and healthsite educational programs (e.g., Heart At Work, the AHA's prevention and cardiovascular risk-intervention program), the AHA works toward achieving its mission. Also available through the AHA are healthful educational and fundraising activities such as "Dance for Heart" and "Heart Challenge."

Centers for Disease Control & Prevention (CDC)
4770 Bufford Hwy. N.E., MS-K46
Atlanta, GA 30341
Phone 770-488-5449
www.cdc.gov

The Centers for Disease Control and Prevention is recognized as the lead federal agency for protecting the health and safety of individuals at home and abroad, providing credible information to enhance health decisions, and promoting health through strong partnerships. The CDC serves as the national focus for developing and applying disease prevention and control, environmental health, and health promotion and education activities designed to improve the health and well-being of Americans.

Cooper Institute for Aerobics Research
12330 Preston Rd.
Dallas, TX 75230
Phone 972-341-3200, Fax 1-800-635-7050
www.cooperinst.org

The Cooper Institute conducts research in epidemiology, exercise physiology, behavior change, hypertension, children's health issues, obesity, nutrition, aging, and other health issues. Research papers from the Cooper Institute are among the most frequently cited references in the scientific literature on topics related to physical fitness, physical activity, and health. The Cooper Institute also offers a variety of training and certification programs for health and fitness professionals.

International Health, Racquet, and Sportsclub Association (IHRSA)
263 Summer St.
Boston, MA 02210
800-228-4772 Fax 617-951-0055
www.ihrsa.org

The International Health, Racquet, and Sportsclub Association is a not-for-profit trade association representing health and fitness facilities, gyms, spas, sportsclubs, and suppliers worldwide. The mission of IHRSA is to grow, protect, and promote the health and fitness industry and to provide its over 6000 members with benefits that will help them be more successful. IHRSA also holds several international trade shows and conventions each year.

The National Association for Health and Fitness
401 West Michigan Street
Indianapolis, IN 46202
317-955-0957
www.physicalfitness.org

The National Association for Health and Fitness is a non-profit organization that exists to improve the quality of life for individuals in the United States through the promotion of physical fitness, sports, and healthy lifestyles, and by supporting the governors' and states' councils on physical fitness and sports.

National Athletic Trainers Association (NATA)
2952 Stemmons Fwy.
Dallas, TX 75247
800-879-6282
www.nata.org

NATA is a voluntary individual membership organization dedicated exclusively to promoting the interests of the athletic training profession, to providing a variety of useful services to athletic trainers, and to serving as resource for information about the practice and profession of athletic training.

National Strength & Conditioning Association (NSCA)
1955 N. Union Blvd.
Colorado Springs, CO 80909
719-632-6722
www.nsca-lift.org

The National Strength & Conditioning Association is a non-profit educational association dedicated to strength and conditioning for improved physical performance and injury reduction. Now in its 21st year of operation, the NSCA has approximately 16,000 members. The NSCA currently offers certifications for two groups of fitness professionals: strength and conditioning specialists and personal trainers.

President's Council on Physical Fitness & Sports (PCPFS)
200 Independence Ave. S.W., Room 738H
Washington, DC 20201
202-690-9000
www.fitness.gov

The President's Council on Physical Fitness & Sports serves as a catalyst to promote, encourage, and motivate Americans of all ages to become physically active and participate in sports. Assisted by elements of the U.S. Public Health Service, the PCPFS advises the President and the Secretary of Health and Human Services on how to encourage more Americans to be physically fit and active.

Wellness Councils of America (WELCOA)
9802 Nicholas St. Ste. 315
Omaha, NE 68114-2106
402-827-3590 Fax 402-827-3594
www.welcoa.org

Wellness Councils of America is a national non-profit membership organization dedicated to promoting healthier lifestyles for all Americans, especially through health promotion activities at the worksite. In addition to helping organizations develop sound wellness programs, WELCOA serves as a national clearinghouse and information center on worksite wellness.

REFERENCE

IDEA. (2001). IDEA Health & Fitness Association's Opinion Statement: Benefits of a Working Relationship Between Medical and Allied Health Practitioners and Personal Fitness Trainers. *IDEA Health & Fitness Source*, September.

NUTRITION

It is now recognized that a lack of nutrition knowledge and poor eating habits can contribute to poor fitness, low energy stores, and the development of such lifestyle-related diseases as heart disease, some types of cancer, and obesity. The time is right for Americans to start making wise food choices and commit to an exercise program. Eating well is not difficult in principle. All that is needed is to eat a selection of foods that supplies appropriate amounts of the essential nutrients and energy. Yet, putting this into practice may be extremely difficult for some. PFTs help fire fighters commit to fitness programs, and guide them in making appropriate food selections for good health. Becoming knowledgeable about nutrition puts you in a position to provide sound, credible nutrition information to your fellow fire fighters in terms they can understand and follow.

NUTRIENTS

Nutrients are life-sustaining substances found in food. There are at least 40 specific nutrients that satisfy three basic needs: energy, tissue growth and repair, and regulation of metabolic functions that are constantly occurring in the body.

CHAPTER

Table 3.1
The Six Classes of Nutrients
and Their Major Functions

Nutrient	Function
Protein	✔ Builds and repairs body tissue ✔ Major component of enzymes, hormones and antibodies
Carbohydrate	✔ Provides a major source of fuel to the body ✔ Provides dietary fibers
Lipids	✔ Chief storage form of energy in the body ✔ Insulate and protect vital organs ✔ Provides dietary fibers
Vitamins	✔ Help promote and regulate various chemical reactions and bodily processes ✔ Do not yield energy themselves, but participate in releasing energy from food
Minerals	✔ Enable enzymes to function ✔ A component of hormones ✔ A part of bone and nerve impulses
Water	✔ Enables chemical reactions to occur ✔ About 60 percent of the body is composed of water ✔ Essential for life as we cannot store it, nor conserve it

Nutrients are divided into classes based on their chemical structure and function. Water, vitamins, minerals, protein, carbohydrates, and fats are the six major classes of nutrients. Table 3.1 lists the nutrient classes and their major functions.

WATER

The most important nutrient, water, is second only to oxygen as essential to sustain life. It is the most abundant substance in the body, accounting for 50 to 70% of the body's weight. All tissues contain varying amounts of water. It makes up 75% of muscle tissue, but only 25% of fat. The body weight of lean individuals is comprised of a relatively high percentage of water. Conversely, the body weight of individuals with a high percentage of body fat is made up of a considerably lower percentage of water.

The body uses water for most of its functions, as every cell in the body relies on water to carry out its activities. Water is required to transport nutrients to and remove wastes from the cells, as well as help to regulate body temperature. Failure to consume adequate water results in fatigue, faulty regulation of body temperature, and increased risk of heat exhaustion and heat stroke. Thirst is not a good indicator of hydration; by the time you feel thirsty you are well on the way to becoming dehydrated. The minimum fluid intake is eight cups a day. It is especially important to stay hydrated when exposed to high temperatures, when dieting, and during exercise.

VITAMINS AND MINERALS

Vitamins are organic substances that are essential to life and play a key role in energy production, growth, maintenance, and repair. Vitamins are only needed in small amounts; they must be obtained from the diet, as the body cannot manufacture them. There are 13 vitamins needed by humans. They provide no calories and, therefore, cannot be used for fuel.

Vitamins are divided into two categories: water-soluble and fat-soluble. Vitamins A, D, E, and K are fat-soluble vitamins that are absorbed with the help of fats, and are stored in fat. There are eight water-soluble vitamins: the B vitamins and vitamin C. Table 3.2 outlines the functions of vitamins as well as common food sources.

Minerals are inorganic substances that must be included in the diet to maintain a number of vital functions and body processes, such as the regulation of heart beat, transportation of oxygen to every cell, formation of hemoglobin, the building of bones and teeth, and muscle contraction. Minerals that are required in amounts greater than 100 milligrams per day may be referred to as major minerals and include calcium, phosphorous, sodium, chloride, and magnesium. Minor minerals needed in smaller amounts, also referred to as trace minerals, include iron, zinc, copper, iodine, manganese, molybdenum, arsenic, boron, nickel, and silicon. The various functions and sources of these minerals are summarized in Table 3.3.

Vitamin and Mineral Supplements: If a Little Is Good, Is More Better?

More is not better when it comes to supplements. Most people do not realize that an upper limit of intake has been established for many nutrients for safety purposes. In fact, continuous over-consumption of many nutrients can result in toxicity and even death. While toxicity from vitamin and mineral supplements is rare, over-supplementing can commonly cause vitamin and mineral interactions that can have a negative influence on health. Keep in mind the following guidelines:

- *Only consume up to, or less than, 10 times the RDA for any vitamin or mineral.* The RDAs (Recommended Dietary Allowances) are nutrient recommendations designed to meet to the need of essentially all people of similar age and gender. The RDAs are a general guide for estimating your nutrient needs. On the back of a supplement label, 10 times the RDA is 1000% intake of that nutrient.

- *Fat-soluble vitamins, especially A, D, and K, are stored in your tissues and are more likely to be harmful when taken in excess.* It is especially important not to consume more than 10 times the RDA daily for these nutrients. The exception is vitamin E, a powerful antioxidant. Leading scientists recommend that adults consume 100–400 IU of vitamin E a day.

- *Minor (trace) minerals are more likely to be toxic in large amounts.*

- *Minerals may compete in the intestine for absorption.* Excessive intake of a single mineral (usually through a large supplemented dose) can restrict the absorption of a competing mineral.

Table 3.2
Vitamin Facts

Vitamin	RDA/AI* Men**	RDA/AI* Women**	Best Sources	Functions
A (carotene)	**900 mcg**	**700 mcg**	yellow or orange fruits and vegetables, green leafy vegetables, fortified oatmeal, liver, dairy products	formation and maintenance of skin, hair, and mucous membranes; helps you see in dim light; bone and tooth growth
B₁ (thiamine)	**1.2mg**	**1.1 mg**	fortified cereals and oatmeals, meats, rice and pasta, whole grains, liver	helps body release energy from carbohydrates during metabolism; growth and muscle tone
B₂ (riboflavin)	**1.3mg**	**1.1 mg**	whole grains, green leafy vegetables, organ meats, milk, eggs	helps body release energy from protein, fat and carbohydrates during metabolism
B₆ (pyridoxine)	**1.3mg**	**1.3mg**	fish, poulty, lean meats, bananas, prunes, dried beans, whole grains, avocados	helps build body tissue and aids in metabolism of protein
B₁₂ (cobalamin)	**2.4mcg**	**2.4mcg**	meats, milk products, seafood	aids cell development, functioning of the nervous system and the metabolism of protein and fat
Biotin	30 mcg	30 mcg	cereal/grain products, yeast, legumes, liver	involved in metabolism of protein, fats, and carbohydrates
Choline	550 mg	425 mg	milk, liver, eggs, peanuts	a precursor of acetylcholine; essential for liver function
Folate (Folacin, folic acid)	**400 mcg**	**400 mcg**	green leafy vegetables, organ meats, dried peas, beans, lentils	aids in genetic material development; involved in red blood cell production
Niacin	**16 mg**	**14 mg**	meat, poultry, fish, enriched cereals, peanuts, potatoes, dairy products, eggs	involved in carbohydrate, protein, and fat metabolism
Pantothenic Acid	5 mg	5 mg	lean meats, whole grains, legumes, vegetables, fruits	helps release energy from fats and carbohydrates
C (absorbic acid)	**90mg**	**75mg**	citrus fruits, berries and vegetables — especially peppers	essential for structure of bones, cartilage, muscle and blood vessels; helps maintain capillaries and gums and aids in absorption of iron
D	5 mcg	5 mcg	fortified milk, sunlight, fish eggs, butter, fortified margarine	aids in bone and tooth formation; helps maintain heart action and nervous system
E	**15 mg**	**15 mg**	fortified and multi-grain cereals, nuts, wheat germ, vegetable oils, green leafy vegetables	protects blood cells, body tissue and essential fatty acids and harmful destruction in the body
K	120 mcg	90 mcg	green leafy vegetables, dairy, grain products	essential for blood-clotting functions

* Recommended Daily Allowances are presented in bold type; Adequate Intakes are presented in ordinary type
** RDAs and AIs given are for men aged 31-50 and non-pregnant, non-breastfeeding women aged 31-50;
   mg = milligrams; mcg = micrograms

Source: Adapted from the following DRI reports, which may be accessed via www.nap.edu: Dietary Reference Intakes for Calcium, Phosphorous, Magnesium, Vitamin D, and Fluoride (1997); Dietary Reference Intakes for Thiamin, Riboflavin, Niacin, Vitamin B6, Folate, Vitamin B12, Pantothenic Acid, Biotin, and Choline (1998); Dietary Reference Intakes for Vitamin C, Vitamin E, Selenium, and Carotenoids (2000); and Dietary Reference Intakes for Vitamin A, Vitamin K, Arsenic, Boron, Chromium, Copper, Iodine, Iron, Manganese, Molybdenum, Nickel, Silicon, Vanadium and Zinc (2001).

Table 3.3
Mineral Facts

Vitamin	RDA/AI* Men**	Women**	Best Sources	Functions
Calcium	1000 mg	1000 mg	milk and milk products	strong bones, teeth, muscle tissue; regulates heart beat, muscle action and nerve function; blood clotting
Chromium	35 mcg	25 mcg	corn oil, clams, whole grain cereals, brewer's yeast	glucose metabolisn (energy); increases effectiveness of insulin
Copper	**900 mcg**	**900 mcg**	oysters, nuts, organ meats, legumes	formation of red blood cells, bone growth and health, works with vitamin C to form elastin
Fluoride	4 mg	3 mg	fluorinated water, teas, marine fish	stimulates bone formation; inhibits or even reverses dental caries
Iodine	**150 mcg**	**150 mcg**	seafood, iodized salt	component of hormone thyroxine, which controls metabolism
Iron	**8 mg**	**18 mg**	meats and organ meats, legumes	hemoglobin formation, improves blood quality, increases resistance to stress and disease
Magnesium	**420 mg**	**320 mg**	nuts, green vegetables, whole grains	acid/alkaline balance; important in metabolism of carbohydrates, minerals, and sugar
Manganese	2.3 mg	1.8 mg	nuts, whole grains, vegetables, fruits	enzyme activation; carbohydrate and fat production; sex hormone production; skeletal development
Molybdenum	**45 mcg**	**45 mcg**	legumes, grain products, nuts	functions as a cofactor for a limited number of enzymes in humans
Phosphorus	**700 mg**	**700 mg**	fish, meat, poultry, eggs, grains	bone development; important in protein, fat, and carbohydrate utilization
Potassium	No RDA		lean meat, vegetables, fruits	fluid balance; controls activity of heart muscle, nervous system, kidneys
Selenium	**55 mcg**	**55 mcg**	seafood, organ meats, lean meats, grains	protects body tissues against oxidative damage from radiation, pollution, and normal metabolic processing
Zinc	**11 mg**	**8 mg**	lean meats, liver, eggs, seafood, whole grains	involved in digestion and metabolism; important in development of reproductive system; aids in healing

See Table 3.2, page 29 for notes and sources.

While it is important not to overuse supplements, vitamin and mineral supplements can be a good complement to the fire fighter's diet if used appropriately. A good supplement regimen for fire fighters is to take a gender-specific multivitamin, 100–400 IU of vitamin E, and 250 mg of vitamin C. Not all vitamin/mineral supplements on the market are the same. Look for the following when making a supplement choice:

1) A toll free number to contact the manufacturer for information about the product you purchased

2) A quality assurance guaranty statement, usually including a statement about the purity of the product (assuring what is on the label is actually in the product)

3) An expiration date (usually month and year)

4) A brand name you recognize (this includes the store's name)

The Caloric Nutrients: Protein, Carbohydrate, and Fat

Proteins, carbohydrates, and fats are the three nutrients that provide calories. A calorie is a way of measuring the potential heat energy in the food we eat. The formal definition of a calorie is the amount of energy expended in raising the temperature of one gram of water one degree Celsius. These calorie sources are used by the body to sustain life by providing all the energy needed by the body to function, including physical muscle movement, maintaining body temperature, and facilitating the growth and repair of all organs and tissues.

Many people believe carbohydrate calories to be "good" calories and fat calories to be "bad" calories. In reality, they are both vital to our diets. One reason fat calories are considered bad is that Americans eat too many of them, which can result in excess body fat and weight. Fat is a very concentrated source of energy and contains more than twice the calories of protein or carbohydrates.

1 gram protein = 4 calories

1 gram carbohydrate = 4 calories

1 gram fat = 9 calories

1 gram alcohol = 7 calories

Alcohol also provides calories, but is not considered a nutrient since it does not contribute to the growth, maintenance, or repair of body tissue. Alcohol can be converted to fat when total caloric intake exceeds caloric expenditure, and it also can be damaging to tissues if consumed in excessive amounts for long periods of time.

PROTEIN

Proteins are organic substances containing carbon, oxygen, hydrogen, and nitrogen. Each protein molecule is made up of subunits called amino acids. Twenty different amino acids are found in the body, 12 of which it can manufacture on its own. The remaining eight amino acids are considered essential and must be consumed through our diet. Table 3.4 lists the protein in common foods.

Meat, fish, poultry, and dairy products contain all of the essential amino acids and are, therefore, considered complete proteins. Vegetables, grains, and nuts do not provide all of the essential amino acids by themselves; however, these incomplete protein foods can be combined to get all of the essential amino acids. Figure 3.1 demonstrates how various vegetable proteins can be combined to create complete proteins.

Protein is the body's major building material. The brain, muscles, skin, hair, and connective tissue are all composed primarily of protein. Protein is needed to make the enzymes and hormones that regulate body processes such as water balance, and are critical components of the immune system.

Table 3.4
Protein in Common Foods

Food	Portion Size	Protein (grams)
Milk (skim, 2%, whole)	1 cup	8
Yogurt (nonfat, lowfat)	1 cup	8
Cheese (any variety)	1 ounce	8
Lean Hamburger Patty	3 ounces	26
Egg/Egg White	1	7
Lean Steak	3 ounces	21
Chicken Breast	3.5 ounces	30
Taco	1	11
Pizza	2 slices	32
Tuna	3 ounces	24
Peanut Butter	1 tablespoon	4
Whole Wheat Bread	1 slice	2
Pasta	1 cup	4

Finally, protein can be used as a source of energy, but only when the diet is limited in carbohydrates and fats. If energy needs are met, excess protein is stored as fat.

The average American diet, often dominated by such foods as steak and eggs, is comprised of too much protein. Because many high-protein foods also are high in fat and calories, this type of diet may encourage weight gain. Still, many people view a high-protein diet as a means of losing weight. The dangers of this type of diet are discussed in detail later in this section.

CARBOHYDRATES

Carbohydrates are the body's best source of energy. As carbohydrate foods make their way through the digestive system, they are broken down into a more usable form of energy called glucose. Glucose is the only form of carbohydrate that the body can use directly for energy and the only energy source used by the brain and nervous system. Glucose can be stored in the liver and muscles where it is transformed to glycogen and used as an energy source during exercise.

Some people avoid eating carbohydrates for fear that they are "fattening." This belief arose from fad diets of the 1970s when people eliminated carbohydrate foods from their diet and lost weight very rapidly. But the lost pounds came mostly from water, not fat. It is no surprise that, when they began to eat carbohydrate foods again, their lost weight returned just as rapidly as it left.

Carbohydrates are divided into two types: complex and simple. Complex carbohydrates (or starches), such as bread, rice, cereal, and potatoes, take longer for the body to break down. These foods also can provide fiber and other vitamins and minerals. Simple sugars, which are rapidly digested and absorbed, are found in foods such as fruit and milk, which provide vitamins and minerals. Most simple sugars consumed by Americans, however, come in the form of soft drinks, cakes, cookies, and candy, and provide little more than calories.

Figure 3.1
Protein complementarity chart.
Adapted from Diet for a Small Planet *by Frances M. Lappe.*

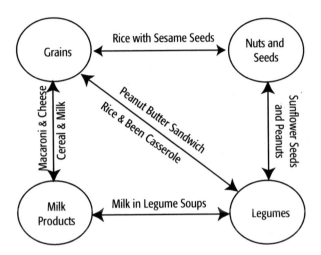

FIBER

Fiber, the indigestible part of a carbohydrate, makes up the cell wall of all plant foods. Fiber is an important element of a healthy diet. Fibers are grouped into two categories: insoluble and soluble. Insoluble fibers are composed of cellulose and add bulk to the diet. Soluble fibers form gels in water and are composed primarily of pectin and guar gums. Both types are important because of their distinct health benefits. Soluble fiber may help reduce blood cholesterol and blood glucose in some people, while insoluble fiber is important for proper bowel function, and can reduce symptoms of chronic constipation, diverticular disease, and hemorrhoids. Most fiber-containing foods have a combination of both types of fibers. Good sources of fiber include whole grain/wheat foods, fruits, vegetables, and legumes/beans.

A high-fiber diet (25 to 35 grams of fiber per day) may help to reduce the risk of heart disease, cancer, diabetes, and diverticular disease. High-fiber foods help control weight, because fiber swells in the stomach; this gives people a more satisfied and full feeling after eating. Most people only eat about one-half the recommended intake for fiber. When increasing fiber intake, do so gradually and drink plenty of water.

FAT

For many years, researchers have repeatedly found that high-fat diets are associated with heart disease. Unfortunately, the implications of these findings have led to a nationwide fear of fat, making it the most misunderstood of all essential nutrients. Fat is a source of energy, supplying the fatty acids necessary for many of the body's activities. Linoleic acid, for example, is an essential fatty acid that must come from the diet and is needed to ensure proper growth in children and to make hormones and cell membranes. This essential polyunsaturated fat is found in vegetable oils, nuts, seeds, and wheat germ. Fats are essential for carrying the fat-soluble vitamins into the body, and enhance the flavor, aroma, and texture of foods. Only a small amount of fat – as little as one tablespoon a day of polyunsaturated fat – is needed to meet our basic nutritional needs. While experts recommend that we eat more than this, they also recommend that we limit fat intake to no more than 30% of our total calories. People who are trying to lose weight may limit their fat intake to as little as 20% of total calories.

Fat and Cholesterol

For years, people were taught that they simply needed to eat less cholesterol to reduce serum cholesterol. It was then found that the amount and type of fat consumed influenced blood cholesterol levels more than the amount of dietary cholesterol consumed. Food companies and health professionals discuss fats in terms of "good" fats and "bad" fats, because the two types affect cholesterol carriers in different ways. Good fats are the polyunsaturated and monounsaturated fats (fats from plant sources), and bad fats are the saturated fats (fats from animal sources). In reality, most dietary fats contain varying amounts of all three types (Figure 3.2).

Figure 3.2
A comparison of dietary fats

		Dietary Cholesterol (MG/TBSP)	% Saturated Fat	% Poly-unsaturated Fat	% Mono-unsaturated Fat	
Comparison of Dietary Fats						
Type	Dietary Fat					
M	Canola oil	0	6	32	62	Vegetable Fats
P	Safflower oil	0	10	77	13	
P	Sunflower oil	0	11	69	20	
P	Corn oil	0	13	62	25	
M	Olive oil	0	14	9	77	
P	Soybean oil	0	15	61	24	
M	Peanut oil	0	18	33	49	
S	Chicken fat	11	31	22	47	Animal Fats
S	Lard	12	41	12	47	
S	Beef fat	14	52	4	44	
S	Butter	33	66	4	30	

Legend: M= Monounsaturated fat   P= Polyunsaturated fat   S = Saturated fat   *Source: U.S. Department of Agriculture*

Saturated fats generally come from animal sources (meats, dairy products) and are solid at room temperature. Other non-animal sources of saturated fat include tropical oils such as coconut and palm kernel oil. Saturated fats interfere with the removal of cholesterol from the blood.

Polyunsaturated fats come from plant sources and are liquid at room temperature. Examples include corn, safflower, and sunflower oils. They tend to lower cholesterol in the blood by lowering the level of low-density lipoproteins (LDLs), those responsible for depositing cholesterol onto the artery walls. One drawback to polyunsaturated fats is that they also lower the level of high-density lipoproteins (HDLs), the so-called good cholesterol.

Monounsaturated fats also are liquid at room temperature and are found in peanut, canola, and olive oils. These fats reduce total blood cholesterol by lowering the LDL fraction while keeping the HDL stable.

The National Cholesterol Education Program recommends keeping blood cholesterol levels at less than 200 mg/dl, with HDL and LDL levels greater than 40 mg/dl and less than 100 mg/dl, respectively. It is important that fire fighters know not only their total cholesterol, but also their HDL, which is responsible for carrying cholesterol to the liver for removal. To help achieve this goal, keep total fat intake to less than 30% of all calories, and choose fats that are high in monounsaturated fat (peanut, canola, and olive oils) rather than saturated fat (animal fat).

PUTTING IT TOGETHER: A HEALTHY MEAL PLAN

WHY IS IT SO HARD TO MAKE WISE FOOD CHOICES?

Why are we so tempted to eat foods that we know we should avoid? What triggers our eating habits? Why do we like high-fat, high-calorie foods? Many factors influence our eating patterns, including hunger, habits, economics, marketing, availability, convenience, and nutritional value. Probably the strongest reason we choose to eat certain foods is for taste. We like the taste of sweet and salty foods and, as a result, we tend to eat too many of them. We also like foods that have happy associations, such as those we eat at family gatherings or on holidays. Social pressure has a very powerful influence on food choices and is evident in every culture and social circle. Many of us have been programmed to feel that it is rude not to accept food in certain social situations, and we've all felt the pressure of eating at work, even though we are not hungry or are trying to watch caloric intake. Availability, convenience, and economics each play a role in choosing foods. You cannot eat foods that are unavailable or unaffordable. In addition, because we are all so busy, we tend to pick foods based on convenience. We are more likely to choose foods that we can pop in the microwave and eat in five minutes, than take the time to prepare a meal from scratch. Both physical and emotional stresses affect our eating habits. Some people respond to stress, whether positive or negative, by eating; others may use food to ward off boredom or anxiety.

So, there are a variety of reasons for choosing the foods we do. How do you get your peers, and perhaps yourself, to select foods with good nutritional value? Knowledge of the nutritional value of food, combined with guidelines for meal planning, will help you successfully teach others how to eat foods that are satisfying while supplying them with adequate amounts of nutrients for optimal health and fitness. To help people make good food decisions, the U.S. Department of Agriculture has established the Dietary Guidelines and Food Guide Pyramid.

DIETARY GUIDELINES*

The Dietary Guidelines issued by the U.S. Department of Agriculture and the Department of Health and Human Services were revised in 2005. They provide science-based recommendations to promote health and reduce risk for major chronic diseases (e.g., cardiovascular disease, type 2 diabetes, hypertension, osteoporosis, certain cancers) through proper diet and physical activity. Revised every five years, the Dietary Guidelines summarize current scientific knowledge of individual nutrients and food components into recommendations for a pattern of eating that can be adopted by the public. Implemented as a whole, the Dietary Guidelines encourage most Americans to eat fewer calories, become more physically active, and make wiser food choices.

The 2005 edition of the Dietary Guidelines are as follows:

1. *Consume adequate nutrients within calorie needs.* Balanced eating patterns such as those described in the USDA MyPyramid Food Guidance System and the Dietary Approaches to Stop Hypertension (DASH) Eating Plan help individuals consume a variety of nutrient-dense foods that limit the intake of saturated and trans fats, cholesterol, added sugars, salt, and alcohol. Both eating patterns provide energy intake recommendations across a range of calorie levels to meet the needs of various age and gender groups (Tables 3.5–3.8). These eating patterns are not promoted as weight-loss diets, rather they are examples of how to eat in accordance with the Dietary Guidelines.

2. *Promote weight management.* Adults should strive to maintain a healthy body weight by balancing calories consumed with calories expended. Those who need to lose weight should aim for slow, steady weight loss by decreasing calorie intake and increasing physical activity.

3. *Incorporate physical activity.* New to the Dietary Guidelines in 2005 is the addition of specific physical activity recommendations for different population groups. Adults who desire to lower their risk of chronic disease should engage in at least 30 minutes of moderate-intensity physical activity most days of the week. Although regular participation in 30 minutes of moderate-intensity exercise promotes health and psychological well-being, most people will receive greater health benefits by engaging in activities of more vigorous intensity for longer durations. Engaging in approximately 60 minutes of moderate- to vigorous-intensity physical activity on most days of the week while not exceeding caloric requirements will help adults manage body weight and help prevent gradual weight gain. For adults who have lost weight, 60 to 90 minutes of daily moderate-intensity exercise while not exceeding caloric intake require-

---

* Reprinted from the *ACE Personal Trainer Manual* (2005) with permission of the American Council on Exercise.

ments may help to sustain previous weight-loss achievements. Other recommendations include guidelines for children and adolescents (engage in at least 60 minutes of physical activity on most days of the week) and older adults (participate in regular exercise to reduce functional declines associated with aging).

4. *Emphasize the consumption of certain food groups.* Daily consumption of a variety of fruits and vegetables, whole grains, and non-fat or low-fat dairy products within caloric intake requirements is recommended. For example, individuals at the 2,000 calorie per day level are advised to consume 2 cups of fruit, 2.5 cups of vegetables, 3 or more ounce-equivalents of whole-grain products, and 3 cups of fat-free or low-fat milk products daily.

5. *Select the appropriate fats.* Total fat intake should range between 20–35% of daily calories, with most fats coming from polyunsaturated and monounsaturated sources (e.g., fish, nuts, vegetable oils). Consuming lean meats and poultry, dry beans, and low-fat or fat-free dairy products is recommended for ensuring adequate protein intake without increasing unhealthy (saturated) fat intake. In addition, no more than 10% of calories should come from saturated fats and consuming less than 300 mg per day of cholesterol is advised. Products containing trans fatty acids should be limited or avoided.

6. *Select the appropriate carbohydrates.* Fiber-rich fruits, vegetables, and whole grains represent the majority of carbohydrate consumption in a healthy diet. Foods and beverages that contain little added sugars or caloric sweeteners should be chosen and prepared. Limiting sugar- and starch-containing foods and beverages along with good oral hygiene will help to reduce the incidence of dental caries.

7. *Balance sodium and potassium consumption.* Americans are advised to choose and prepare foods with little salt and to limit consumption to less than 2,300 mg of sodium (approximately 1 teaspoon of salt) per day. Potassium-rich foods, such as fruits and vegetables, should be consumed daily in the amounts recommended by the USDA MyPyramid Food Guidance System and the DASH Eating Plan.

8. *Limit alcoholic beverage intake.* Sensible and moderate consumption of alcoholic beverages—defined as no more than one drink per day for women and no more than two drinks per day for men—is recommended. Certain individuals, such as women of childbearing age who may become pregnant, pregnant and lactating women, children and adolescents, individuals taking medication that may interact with alcohol, and those with specific medical conditions should avoid alcoholic beverages. Furthermore, individuals planning to drive or operate machinery should avoid consuming alcohol.

9. *Enhance food safety.* The incidence of microbial food-borne illness may be limited or prevented by practicing the following key recommendations for handling food. Hands, food contact surfaces, and fruits and vegetables should be cleaned prior to food preparation. Raw, cooked, and read-to-eat foods should be separated from each

other while shopping, preparing, or storing them. Foods should be cooked to a safe temperature and perishable foods should be refrigerated and/or defrosted properly. Unpasteurized milk products and juices, raw eggs and sprouts, or undercooked or raw meats and poultry should be avoided.

THE MYPYRAMID FOOD GUIDANCE SYSTEM

The MyPyramid Food Guidance System (Figure 3.3) provides food-based guidance to help implement the recommendations of the 2005 Dietary Guidelines for Americans. MyPyramid provides specific recommendations for making food choices that will improve the quality of an average American diet as it translates the Dietary Guidelines into a total diet that meets nutrient needs from food sources. If followed properly, MyPyramid results in the following changes to a typical diet:

- Increased intake of vitamins, minerals, dietary fiber, and other essential nutrients through increased consumption of fruits, vegetables, and whole-grains

- Lowered intake of saturated fats, trans fats, and cholesterol

- Calorie intake balanced with energy needs to prevent weight gain and/or promote a healthy weight

There are six general topic areas presented in the MyPyramid Food Guidance System. The topics represent a personalized approach to eating and physical activity and are meant to

Figure 3.3
The MyPyramid Food Guidance System.

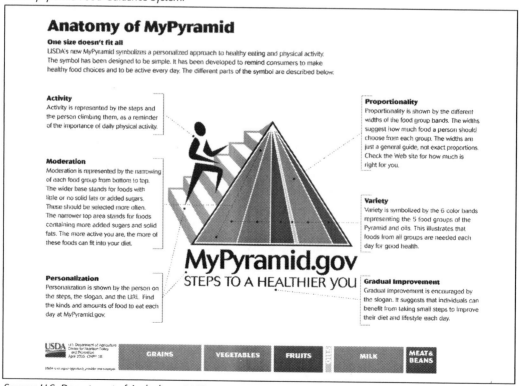

Source: U.S. Department of Agriculture, 2005

remind consumers to make healthy food choices and be active every day. First, MyPyramid emphasizes daily physical activity which is represented by the person climbing the steps on the left side of the pyramid. The second topic is moderation and is symbolized by the narrowing of each food group from the bottom of the pyramid to the top. The wider base stands for food selections with little or no saturated and trans fats or added sugars. The narrower top portion of the pyramid stands for foods containing more added sugars and solid fats that should be limited in the typical diet. Personalization is the third topic and can be applied by understanding the kinds and amounts of food to eat each day based on an individual's age, gender, and activity level. Proportionality, the fourth topic is shown by the different widths of the food groups displayed in the pyramid. The widths suggest the relative amount of food one should select from each group. For example, the food groups represented by larger widths (i.e., grains, vegetables, fruits, milk) should be consumed in relatively larger amounts than the food groups represented by smaller widths (i.e., meat and beans, oils). The fifth topic, variety, suggests that individuals eat foods from all food groups daily. Variety is symbolized by the six different colored stripes that make up the pyramid. Finally, the sixth topic, gradual improvement, implies that improvements in diet and lifestyle are best achieved by taking small steps daily. For the average person, preventing gradual weight gain over time or improving current health status involves making small decreases in calorie intake and moderate increases in physical activity.

Table 3.5
Sample USDA Food Guide and the DASH Eating Plan at the 2,000-Calorie Level[1]

Food Groups & Subgroups	USDA Food Guide Amount[2]	DASH Eating Plan Amount
Fruit Group	2 cups (4 servings)	2 to 2.5 cups (4 to 5 servings)
Vegetable Group	2.5 cups (5 servings)	2 to 2.5 cups (4 to 5 servings)
• Dark green vegetables	• 3 cups/week	
• Orange vegetables	• 2 cups/week	
• Legumes (dry beans)	• 3 cups/week	
• Starchy vegetables	• 3 cups/week	
• Other vegetables	• 6.5 cups/week	
Grain Group	6 ounce-equivalents	7 to 8 ounce-equivalents
• Whole grains	• 3 ounce-equivalents	(7 to 8 servings)
• Other grains	• 3 ounce-equivalents	
Meat & Beans Group	5.5 ounce-equivalents	• 6 ounces or less: meat, poultry and fish
		• 4 to 5 servings per week: nuts, seeds and dry beans[3]
Milk Group	3 cups	2 to 3 cups
Oils	24 grams (6 tsp)	8 to 12 grams (2 to 3 tsp)
Discretionary Calorie Allowance	267 calories	
• Example of distribution:		
Solid fat[4]	18 grams	~ 2 tsp (5 Tbsp per week)
Added sugars	8 tsp	

[1] All servings are per day unless otherwise noted. USDA vegetable subgroup amounts and amounts of DASH nuts, seeds, and dry beans are per week.

[2] The 2,000-calorie USDA Food Guide is appropriate for many sedentary males 51 to 70 years of age, sedentary females 19 to 30 years of age, and for some other gender/age groups who are more physically active.

[3] In the DASH Eating Plan, nuts, seeds and dry beans are a separate food group from meat, poultry and fish.

[4] The oils listed in this table are not considered to be part of discretionary calories because they are a major source of the vitamin E and polyunsaturated fatty acids, including the essential fatty acids, in the food pattern. In contrast, solid fats (i.e., saturated and trans fats) are listed separately as a source of discretionary calories.

SOURCE: United States Department of Agriculture, 2005

Table 3.6
Daily Amount of Food from Each Group

Calorie Level[1]	1,600	1,800	2,000	2,200
Fruits[2]	1.5 cups	1.5 cups	2 cups	2 cups
Vegetables	2 cups	2.5 cups	2.5 cups	3 cups
Grains	5 oz-eq	6 oz-eq	6 oz-eq	7 oz-eq
Meat and Beans	5 oz-eq	5 oz-eq	5.5 oz-eq	6 oz-eq
Milk	3 cups	3 cups	3 cups	3 cups
Oils	5 tsp	5 tsp	6 tsp	6 tsp
Discretionary Calorie Allowance	132	195	267	290

[1] A wider range of calorie levels (1,000–3,200) is available on www.mypyramid.gov. See Table 8.7 for help in assigning individuals to the food intake patterns at particular calorie levels.

[2] See www.mypyramid.gov for information on each of the food groups and tips for reaching these amounts for each calorie level.

SOURCE: United States Department of Agriculture, 2005

Table 3.7
Vegetable Subgroup Amounts Per Week

Calorie Level[1]	1,600	1,800	2,000	2,200
Dark green vegetables	2 cups	3 cups	3 cups	3 cups
Orange vegetables	1.5 cups	2 cups	2 cups	2 cups
Legumes	2.5 cups	3 cups	3 cups	3 cups
Starchy vegetables	2.5 cups	3 cups	3 cups	6 cups
Other vegetables	5.5 cups	6.5 cups	6.5 cups	7 cups

[1] A wider range of calorie levels (1,000–3,200) is available on www.mypyramid.gov.

SOURCE: United States Department of Agriculture, 2005

Table 3.8
Estimated Daily Calorie Needs

Children	Calorie Range Sedentary → Active[1]	Males	Calorie Range Sedentary → Active[1]
2–3 years	1,000 → 1,400	4–8 years	1,400 → 2,000
Females		9–13 years	1,800 → 2,600
4–8 years	1,200 → 1,800	14–18 years	2,200 → 3,200
9–13 years	1,600 → 2,200	19–30 years	2,400 → 3,000
14–18 years	1,800 → 2,400	31–50 years	2,200 → 3,000
19–30 years	2,000 → 2,400	51+	2,000 → 2,800
31–50 years	1,800 → 2,200		
51+	1,600 → 2,200		

[1] Sedentary = a lifestyle that includes only the light physical activity associated with typical day-to-day life; Active = a lifestyle that includes physical activity equivalent to walking more than 3 miles per day at 3 to 4 miles per hour, in addition to the light physical activity associated with typical day-to-day life.

SOURCE: United States Department of Agriculture, 2005

GUIDELINES FOR NUTRITION DECISIONS

Counseling fire fighters to make good nutrition decisions starts with educating them about what they are buying. At restaurants, foods fried or served in a cream sauce have a higher amount of fat and calories and deliver fewer nutrients. Foods sautéed, baked, broiled, or served with a red or vegetable sauce are usually better choices. Table 3.9 provides a list of good menu choices for eating out.

Table 3.9
Discover Nutrition Anytime, Anywhere

Does eating on the run put a detour in your healthy eating plans? Consider your options before grabbing those empty calories. Make your best choice based on what's available. Here are some suggested food choices to get you on the road to good nutrition… anytime, anywhere!

Fast Food
Small hamburger
Baked potato
Salad/reduced-fat dressing
Grilled chicken sandwich
Roast beef sandwich
Roasted chicken
Baked fish
Taco
Fajita

Salad Bar
Raw vegetables
Chick peas/kidney beans
Fresh fruit
Cottage cheese
Diced ham
Marinated mushrooms/beets
Bean salad
Reduced-calorie dressing

Cafeteria
Salad/reduced-fat dressing
Pasta with tomato sauce
Yogurt
Chili

Breakfast/Brunch
Cereal
Bagel
English muffin
Fresh fruit or juice
Waffle
Pancakes
Blueberry or bran muffin
Yogurt

Vending Machine
Pretzels
Raisins/dried fruit
Fruit juice
Trail mix
Crackers with peanut butter
Fig bar cookie
Gingersnaps

Mall
Soft pretzel
Frozen yogurt
Stuffed baked potato
Vegetable pizza slice
Plain popcorn
Tostada chips with salsa

Deli
Turkey breast, smoked
  turkey, ham or roast beef
  on whole wheat bread,
  sub roll, or pita
Grilled chicken salad
Vegetable soup
Vinegar-based coleslaw

Source: National Center for Nutrition and Dietetics of The American Dietetic Association and its Foundation

Once a food is in the firehouse, it is much more difficult to avoid it or eat in moderate amounts. The best way for many people to avoid eating certain foods is to limit access to them by not having them around. This strategy works best at the point of purchase — the grocery store. Other effective strategies are to make a list of what will be purchased before going grocery shopping and avoid shopping when hungry.

Learning to read labels will help those you are counseling make better food choices. The new food label includes a "Nutrition Facts" section that provides consistency and detail, and helps in understanding the value of the food eaten (Figure 3.4). Real-life serving sizes are now more the rule than the exception. The Percent Daily Value has replaced the Percent Recommended Dietary Allowance (RDA) on the new label. The Percent Daily Value helps people know whether an item has a significant amount of a particular nutrient based on a 2,000-

calorie diet. This must be adjusted if intake is more or less than 2,000 calories. For example, if a label reads 10 grams of fat, it would provide 15% of the recommended amount for a 2,000-calorie diet. For a 1,500-calorie diet, it would provide 20% of the Daily Value. The following suggestions illustrate examples of what to look for on labels:

- Foods that have less than 3 g of fat per 100 calories (less than 30% fat)

- Foods that have less than 1 g of saturated fat per 100 calories (less than 10% saturated fat)

- Foods that have at least 2.5 g of fiber per serving

- Foods that have a higher amount of vitamins A and C and minerals calcium and iron

- Foods that are lower in sodium and cholesterol

- Foods that do not list sugar or corn syrup as a first ingredient

Figure 3.4
How to read the new food label.

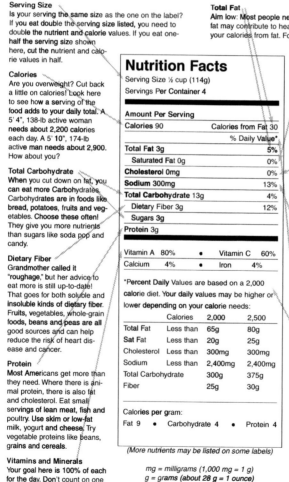

Source: American Heart Association

FAD DIETS

Here is a simple fact: to lose one pound of fat, a fire fighter must under-eat or over-exercise 3,500 calories worth of energy. This is the equivalent of the amount of food an average person needs for two entire days, or the amount of energy burned on a 30-mile run. Losing weight faster than it takes to burn off 3,500 calories results in loss of muscle, water, or stored energy (glycogen), not only fat. Although many diet books try to sell a different story, there really is no shortcut for long-term weight loss.

So if the dieting truths are really myths, why is selling diet programs and supplements a multibillion-dollar industry? Because Americans are over-fat and getting fatter, and everyone would like to believe that weight control could be as easy as taking a pill or following a McDonald's-only meal plan, rather than making some changes in the way we eat. That is not to say that the diet programs out there do not have redeeming features. But it is important to be able to analyze the thinking behind the diet plans and learn the value of healthy eating.

This section will take a look at common diets to give you the facts behind the programs and help you counsel fire fighters to make good nutrition decisions.

HIGH-PROTEIN, LOW-CARBOHYDRATE DIETS

(Dr. Atkins New Diet Revolution, The Carbohydrate Addict's Life-Span Program, Protein Power, Sugar Busters)

Claims

These diet books claim that carbohydrates make you fat by increasing the hormone insulin, which will in turn cause health problems such as heart disease, diabetes, and weight gain. Further, to reduce cravings for carbohydrate foods, you must first reduce or eliminate them from your diet. Meals and snacks should be low in carbohydrate and high in fat and protein.

Facts

High-protein, low-carbohydrate diets have been around since 1967. They are neither "new" nor "revolutionary." Being overweight is rarely the *result* of insulin imbalances. Rather, being over-weight often *causes* problems with insulin and glucose metabolism. Further, there are true health concerns about these diets. Reducing carbohydrates to less than 50 to 100g per day caus-es the body to produce ketones for energy, which strains the kidneys and increases risks of dehydration and electrolyte imbalance. High-protein, low-carbohydrate diets also increase the risk of fatigue, constipation, headaches, and nausea.

People tend to drop weight fast on these diets. However, the weight they are losing at first is not fat weight, but rather water, protein, and muscle glycogen. Continued weight loss is the result of fewer calories eaten, not because of any magic from eating protein.

Redeeming Points

Protein and fat help to make us feel more satisfied from the food we eat. The lesson from the popularity of these diets is to make sure that snacks and meals are not just fat or sugar, but also include protein for more staying power and balance.

Bottom Line

The goal for any diet plan should be improving health, not making it worse. High-protein, low-carbohydrate diets are of special concern for fire fighters because they deplete muscles' primary fuel for high-intensity exercise—glycogen from carbohydrates—and could lead to fatigue. Ketones produced from a low-carbohydrate diet promote dehydration and electrolyte imbalance. Complex carbohydrates provide nutrients, fiber, and energy, and are a critical dietary component for people with high physical demands.

FOOD-SPECIFIC DIETS

(Eat Right 4 Your Type, The New Beverly Hills Diet, The New Cabbage Soup Diet)

Claims

Certain foods have special properties that can cause weight loss or interact in our body in a special way. By eating one type of food only, weight loss results.

Facts

No food can cause weight loss. People lose weight on these diets because eating any food to the exclusion of others will cause you to eat less from boredom. People naturally have an appetite for different foods to ensure that we have a variety of nutrients in our diet.

Redeeming Points

Many of these diets recommend eating wholesome foods, but even wholesome foods should never be eaten at the exclusion of other foods.

Bottom Line

These diets often misrepresent "scientific" information and are not nutritionally sound. Eventually, people become bored with these diets and start craving the foods not on the diet.

LIQUID, LOW-CALORIE, AND FASTING DIETS

Claims

Proponents of these regimens claim that extremely low caloric intake or fasting has beneficial effects including weight loss. Liquid protein diets claim to "spare" protein sources in the body (muscles) from metabolism when fasting for an extended period of time.

Facts

Few individuals can stay on a regimen that requires such drastic changes in eating patterns, according to the American Heart Association. It is unlikely that these dieters are successful in keeping the weight off because they do not learn to change their eating pattern.

Redeeming Points

Weight loss is achieved whenever calorie consumption is restricted; it is simply very difficult to sustain such severe restrictions.

Bottom Line

Reducing caloric intake is the best way to lose weight. However, reducing your caloric intake by too much, too fast may work against you. With most liquid diets, weight plateaus after about three months. On very low-calorie diets, eating below the basal energy expenditure (BEE)—the energy required to keep the body going—will cause metabolism to slow down, further sabotaging weight loss efforts; the individual eats less, but the weight comes off slower.

There are some people that are able to sustain long-term weight loss from eating a reduced calorie diet with a liquid nutritional supplement. Many who attempt such a regime do not feel satisfied from their diet and replacing meals with liquid substitutes does not encourage healthful eating.

WEIGHT MANAGEMENT

There are weight loss programs that promote good health and account for the fact that different programs work for different people. The truth is that for most people, the best way to maintain a healthy body weight is to eat more wholesome, unprocessed foods, limit portions, and eat less high-calorie, high-sugar, high-fat snacks and beverages. These small changes continue to have the largest impact on improving health.

NUTRITION FOR ACTIVITY

From as far back as the ancient Olympians to today's athletes, every imaginable diet has been used to influence performance. As early as 776 BC, athletes and trainers knew what science is proving today: proper diet choices are critical to optimal physical performance. Incorporating good nutrition principles into training can help decrease body fat, increase muscle mass, improve endurance, reduce injuries, and improve overall health. Defining "proper nutrition," however, is still controversial and athletes, always looking for a performance edge, are often the targets of nutrition misinformation.

Sports nutrition is the application of nutrition principles to enhance sport performance. As a relatively new area of science, sports nutrition is an umbrella term often used for nutrition that relates to physical movement and exercise. Unfortunately, information is often misreported or misinterpreted. Athletes and trainers are bombarded with conflicting recommendations regarding sport-specific nutrient intakes. In addition, science has not kept pace with the rapid introduction of sports supplements and ergogenic aids, making it difficult to know what to do or recommend. Although frustrating, it is important to recognize, and help others recognize, when a diet regime or product could pose more harm than good. This chapter will serve as a foundation for that information.

NUTRITION CONSIDERATIONS TO SUPPORT EXERCISE

The quantity and the quality of the food we eat will affect exercise performance, training response, and overall health. There are six general classes of nutrients, with each nutrient class having specific health functions. These nutrient classes can be separated into those that provide energy for exercise directly (protein, carbohydrates, and fat) and those that indirectly support energy metabolism and other metabolic processes. All six classes of nutrients are vital for optimal training and performance.

There are four primary areas for applying sports nutrition information:

- Energy requirements

- Adequate intake of essential nutrients

- Nutrient intake before, during, and after exercise

- Balance of nutrients

ENERGY

Energy, simply defined, is the ability to do work. We extract energy from the foods we eat, specifically from the nutrient classes we call the macronutrients: protein, carbohydrates, and fat. Energy from carbohydrate, protein, and fat is not automatically released to support muscle contraction and physical exercise. Rather, the food we eat, through a series of complex chemical reactions, is converted into heat energy to fuel work. Calories, a measure of heat, represent the energy value of food. The words energy and calories are often used interchangeably.

About 40% of the energy from food is converted into adenosine triphosphate (ATP, the universal carrier of energy) and used by the muscle to support exercise. We have a very limited amount of stored ATP for energy – about 3 to 4 ounces (1 to 4 seconds of exercise) in a typical person – so it is critical that the body continue to produce ATP when needed. Stored ATP will support energy demands of only a couple of seconds upon the start of exercise. Muscles then incorporate a second energy source, phosphocreatine.

Up to about 20 seconds, phosphocreatine supports ATP production by a transfer of a high-energy phosphate bond. After the phosphocreatine energy reserve is used up, muscles generate ATP from the macronutrients either aerobically (with oxygen) from fat and carbohydrate stores, or anaerobically (without oxygen) using mostly carbohydrate. A limited amount of protein can also support the energy demands of some types of exercise, such as long, endurance events and heavy resistance training.

After 20 to 45 seconds, anaerobic glucose metabolism supports energy needs (producing lactic acid), and after 2 minutes, aerobic glucose metabolism supports energy needs. Note that most physical activities rely on more than one energy generating system, and there is often an overlap of the fuels used (Figure 3.5).

The proportion of anaerobic versus aerobic metabolism depends on the intensity and length of exercise. When the body is working at low exercise intensities, there is more oxygen available and the body can use its aerobic energy systems to metabolize carbohydrate and fat. As the intensity increases, the oxygen needs increase beyond the body's ability to provide it and the oxidation (burning) of carbohydrates increases dramatically. As the intensity of your workout increases to its maximum point, caloric burn is very high (> 10 kcals/min) and most of the energy comes from carbohydrate.

During high-intensity exercise and long-duration exercise, muscles eventually use up their glycogen (stored carbohydrate) stores and become exhausted. In the absence of glycogen, muscles get a greater proportion of their energy from fat and amino acids. Exercise increases the conversion of fats and amino acids to energy in an effort to sustain stored muscle glycogen. A key concept of sports nutrition is to support exercise by delaying fatigue. This is done through exercise conditioning, which improves the efficiency of muscle nutrient use, and through diet to ensure that the nutrients needed to support exercise are available in optimal amounts.

Understanding and supporting the energy requirements of exercise is critical to ensuring the best result from training. Consuming insufficient calories results in insufficient energy to fuel exercise and, ultimately, diminished results from training.

Figure 3.5
Three energy systems and their percentage contribution to total energy output during all-out exercise of different durations.

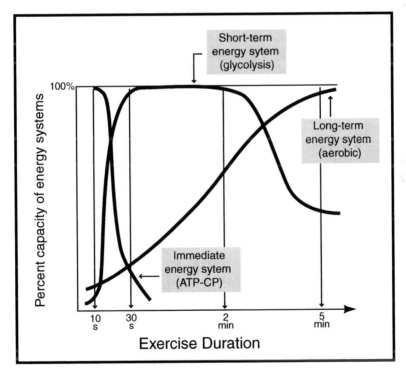

Source: McArdle, W.D., Katch, F.I., & Katch, V.L. (2000). Essentials of Exercise Physiology, 2/e. Philadelphia: Lippincott, Williams & Wilkins

COMPONENTS TO ENERGY REQUIREMENTS

Three components contribute to overall energy needs: basal metabolic rate, physical activity, and the thermic effect of food. Energy (calorie) requirements are unique to each individual.

BASAL METABOLIC RATE (BMR)

BMR is the amount of energy needed to support vital life functions like breathing and keeping your heart beating. It accounts for the largest component to energy needs . The biggest determinant of BMR is lean body mass. Lean body mass is more metabolically active than fat tissue, so it requires more energy to sustain it. About 70 to 80% of BMR is dependent on lean body mass.

The other factors that determine BMR, specifically age and sex, are also related to lean body mass. Males have about 10 to 20% more muscle than females. Since muscle burns more energy than fat, males generally have a 5 to 10% higher BMR as compared to women. Calorie needs peak at about age 25, and begin to decline by about 2% every 10 years. So if at age 25, you need 2200 calories to maintain your weight, you will only need 2110 calories by the age of 45. Other genetic factors influence BMR, such as height and body shape.

PHYSICAL ACTIVITY

Activity is the most variable component to energy needs. The type, intensity, and duration of exercise influences energy expenditure from that exercise. The weight of the person performing the sport also influences calorie expenditure.

While most people assume that exercise is the largest component of an individual's energy needs, usually activity only accounts for 15 to 30% of energy needs. For elite athletes, however, physical activity can actually become a larger component to total energy needs than BMR.

THERMIC EFFECT OF FOOD (TEF)

There is an energy cost for the breakdown, absorption, and use of the food we eat. TEF accounts for about 10% of energy needs. For example, if you eat 2000 calories a day, the TEF would be 200 calories. Some calculations for energy requirements use TEF, while others do not.

Table 3.10 Simple Method of Estimating Resting Metabolic Rate (RMR) and Daily Caloric Needs

---

RMR (for men) = Body Weight (in lb) x 11 kcal/lb
RMR (for women) = Body Weight (in lb) x 10 kcal/lb
Daily Caloric Requirement = RMR x Activity Correction Factor (see below)
Activity Correction Factors:
    Relatively Inactive (i.e., exercises less than 2 days per week) = 1.2
    Moderately Active (i.e., exercises 3 - 4 days per week) = 1.5
    Highly Active (i.e., exercises 5 days or more per week) = 1.8
For example, consider a 180-pound male who is highly active:
    RMR = 180 lbs x 11 kcal/lb = 1980 kcal
    Daily Caloric Requirement = 1980 kcal x 1.8 = 3654

ESTIMATION FOR ENERGY REQUIREMENTS

There are many ways to estimate energy needs. The best estimates incorporate body fat percentage, height, gender, age, and activity level. However, there are many easy calculations that provide you with a rough estimate of energy needs. Two of these "quick and easy" calculations are listed in Table 3.10. Keep in mind that these calculations only yield estimates.

ADEQUATE INTAKE OF ESSENTIAL NUTRIENTS

ENERGY NUTRIENTS

Proteins, carbohydrates, and fats – the energy nutrients – provide the fuel to support exercise. Consuming these nutrients in balanced amounts will enhance the physical performance and health of an active adult.

CARBOHYDRATES

Carbohydrates primarily function as a source of energy for red blood cells, the central nervous system, and muscles. Carbohydrate is the primary fuel during exercise and is the body's only fuel source during high-intensity exercise. Therefore, carbohydrates should be the foundation of an athlete's diet, contributing about 60% of total calorie intake. Most athletes fall short of the recommended intake for carbohydrates, consuming less than 50% of their total caloric intake from carbohydrate. This is also true of the U.S. population in general.

Carbohydrates in the body are stored as glycogen in the muscle and the liver. The amount of glycogen available influences the total amount of energy available to do work. Two factors determine the amount of stored carbohydrate available for exercise: diet and fitness level. As an adaptation to exercise, athletes are able to store more glycogen in their muscle. Diet determines the availability of carbohydrates to be stored as glycogen in the muscle and the rate at which the body replenishes depleted glycogen stores after exercise. There is an overwhelming amount of science that shows athletes on high-carbohydrate diets can exercise longer and at greater intensities compared to athletes on low-carbohydrate diets.

Recommendations for carbohydrate intake are often expressed as a percent of total calorie intake, determined by body weight and physical activity (Figure 3.6). A 220-pound weight lifter requires more energy and therefore 2 to 3 times more carbohydrates than a 150-pound person who only occasionally works out. Carbohydrates should provide 60 to 65% of total energy intake. Sixty percent of calorie intake translates to about 450 to 600 grams of carbohydrate per day. Consistent with the recommendations for good health, the majority of those carbohydrates should be complex carbohydrates, such as whole grains, pasta, cereals and vegetables (Table 3.11).

Not only do complex carbohydrates provide energy, they are also packed with nutrients and are good sources of fiber. Simple carbohydrates (sugars) do provide energy, but they provide little additional nutrition.

Figure 3.6 *EXAMPLE: CARBOHYDRATE REQUIREMENT*

<u>220-lb *body builder*</u>

calorie needs = 3,600 kcal/day

carbohydrate = 2,160 kcal or 60% of diet

grams of carbohydrate per day = 540 g

<u>150-lb *recreational athlete*</u>

calorie needs = 2,127 kcal/day

carbohydrate = 1,170 kcal or 55% of diet

grams of carbohydrate per day = 292 g

Table 3.11 Complex and Simple Carbohydrates

COMPLEX CARBOHYDRATES

	SERVING	CALORIES	CARB (GRAMS)
Wheat bread	1 slice	69	13
Bagel, small	2 oz	163	31
Plain pancake	1 small	60	9
Cheerios	1 cup	88	16
Oatmeal	1 cup	145	25
Spaghetti noodles	1 cup	190	39
Baked potato	1 medium	145	34
Rice	1 cup	180	40
Pretzels (hard)	2 large	120	24
Green beans	1 cup	27	6

SIMPLE CARBOHYDRATES

	SERVING	CALORIES	CARB (GRAMS)
Banana	1 medium	81	21
Orange juice	1 cup	62	15
Honey	1 tablespoon	64	16
Sugar	1 tablespoon	46	12
Jelly	1 tablespoon	49	13
Cola drink	12 oz	159	40
Chocolate chip cookie	1 medium	51	6

Source: U.S. Department of Agriculture

Carbohydrate Loading

Muscle glycogen depletion is a well recognized limitation to endurance exercise exceeding 90 minutes. Carbohydrate loading can nearly double an individual's muscle glycogen stores. Obviously, the greater the pre-exercise muscle glycogen, the greater the endurance potential.

The classic study on carbohydrate loading evaluated exercise time to exhaustion. Subjects exercised at 75% $\dot{V}O_2$max after consuming diets with varying amounts of carbohydrates – a low-carbohydrate diet, a normal diet, and a high-carbohydrate diet. The low-carbohydrate diet group sustained only an hour of exercise; the normal diet group 115 minutes of exercise; and the high-carbohydrate diet group sustained 170 minutes of the high-intensity exercise. Following additional research, the carbohydrate loading sequence developed into a week-long regimen, beginning with an exhaustive training session one week before the competition. For the next three days, the athletes consumed low-carbohydrate diets, yet continued exercising to lower muscle glycogen stores even further. Then, for the last three days prior to competition, the athlete rested and consumed a high-carbohydrate diet to promote glycogen supercompensation. For many years, this week-long sequence was considered the optimal way to achieve maximum glycogen storage. However, it has many drawbacks. The three days of reduced carbohydrate intake can cause hypoglycemia (low blood sugar) and ketosis (increased blood acids), which is associated with nausea, fatigue, dizziness, and irritability. These dietary manipulations prove to be too cumbersome for many athletes, and an exhaustive training session the week before competition may predispose athletes to injuries.

A revised method of carbohydrate loading eliminates many of the problems associated with the old regimen. Six days prior to competition, the athlete exercises hard (70 to 75% of aerobic capacity for 90 minutes) and consumes a diet of 60% carbohydrates. On the second and third days, training is decreased to 40 minutes at 70 to 75% aerobic capacity and, the athlete consumes the same 60% carbohydrate diet. On the next two days, the athlete consumes a high-carbohydrate diet providing 70% carbohydrate (about 550 grams, or 10 grams per kg body weight), and reduces training to 20 minutes at 70 to 75% aerobic capacity. On the last day, the athlete rests while maintaining the high-carbohydrate diet. The modified regimen results in muscle glycogen stores equal to that provided by the classic method.

Carbohydrate loading is not fully practiced today, because athletes require maximal glycogen stores every day when they are training. The focus is instead on reducing muscle fatigue caused by repeated daily training by reloading carbohydrate stores everyday. This means that athletes must consume adequate amounts of carbohydrates daily, and take advantage of the faster rate of post-exercise glycogen replenishment by consuming the recommended amount of carbohydrates immediately following exercise.

PROTEIN

Of all the nutrients, protein is the most heavily debated and misunderstood. Protein is made up of a combination of essential amino acids and non-essential amino acids. Our bodies cannot make essential amino acids, so they must be consumed. There are two ways to get all the essential amino acids, either by eating animal proteins (complete proteins) that have all the essential amino acids, or by combining plant proteins.

A common misconception is that protein requirements for the athlete, especially the resistance trained athlete, is much higher than the RDA of 0.8g per kg of body weight. The logic is that large protein servings and protein supplements are needed to support the increased protein demands of training. Protein requirements are higher for an athlete, but this increase in protein requirement is easily met by keeping protein intake, as a percentage of total caloric intake, at 15%. As athletes need higher energy intake to support their muscle mass and training, their diets will proportionately provide them with increased protein to meet their needs (Table 3.12).

Protein is only one of several factors that contribute to increased muscle mass. The largest factor determining body muscle mass results is the amount, intensity, and type of exercise training. Nutritionally, sufficient calorie intake is as important as protein intake. The results of training on muscle development will be much reduced by a calorie deficiency, regardless of how much protein is consumed. The bottom line is that muscle develops by working the muscle, then consuming enough total calories and protein to support the repair and growth of that muscle. There is a limit to how much protein can be used to meet the protein functions in the body. Consuming more protein than is needed results in proteins being used for energy and stored as fat.

Another misconception is that protein supplements are somehow superior to food sources of protein. Actually, our body uses protein from food very efficiently. About 92% of proteins from whole foods are made available to sustain the many functions of protein. Many whole foods provide good amounts of protein per serving (Table 3.13). Protein supplements may be convenient and easier than buying whole foods, but are certainly not superior to whole protein foods for results. Hydrolyzed proteins are very expensive and research has not shown any added benefit from using them.

Table 3.12 EXAMPLE: COMPARISON OF PROTEIN NEEDS

	Body Builder	Cyclist	Non Exerciser
Weight in pounds (lb)	190 lb	190 lb	190 lb
Weight in kilograms (kg)	86.4 kg	86.4 kg	86.4 kg
Calorie needs (calories per day)	3,110 kcal/d	3,110 kcal/d	2,690 kcal/d
Protein needs (grams per kg)	1.6–1.8 g/kg	1.2–1.4 g/kg	0.8 g/kg
Gram (g) amount of protein	138–156 g	104–121 g	69 g
Protein (15% of calorie intake)	155.5 g	116 g	101 g

Table 3.13 Protein Amounts in Whole Foods

FOOD	AMOUNT	CALORIES	PROTEIN GRAMS	FAT GRAMS
Bread	1 slice	80	2–4	0–2
Cereal, Cheerios	1 cup	89	3.4	1.4
Cereal, Bran Flakes	1 cup	152	5.3	0.8
Oatmeal	1 cup	145	6.0	2.0
Cheese	1 slice or 1 oz	107	8	7.5
Cottage Cheese	1/2 cup	109	1	4.8
Egg	1 medium	158	12	11
Tuna, canned in water	4 oz	148	33.4	0.6
Shrimp	4 oz	102	23	2
Milk, skim	1 cup	80	8	<1
Milk, whole	1 cup	142	7.5	7.5
Yogurt, lowfat	1 cup	136	11	2
Chili with red beans	1 cup	220	11	3
Kidney beans	1/2 cup	90	7	<1
Potato	1 large	220	4	0
Pizza Hut Supreme	2 slices	589	32	30
Chicken, light no skin	4 oz	133	27	2
Chicken, dark meat, skin	4 oz	271	19	21

Source: U.S. Department of Agriculture

FAT

The average American consumes about 35% of their calories from fat, and athletes are no different. There is no absolute fat requirement. Current recommendations include keeping fat intake to less than 30% of total calories, and saturated fat (mostly animal fat) to less than 10% of total calories. Many exercise nutritionists suggest keeping fat to less than 25% of total calories for the athletes.

Fat has many important and necessary health functions and is an important component of a healthy diet. Even a lean athlete has an almost unlimited energy reserve from fat. However, there are several factors that limit its use during exercise. First, it takes time (about 20 minutes) for fat to be available for exercise. The energy pathways that make fat available for use by muscles are not as short as those for carbohydrates. Second, fats require carbohydrates to burn completely. Fat burns in a "fire of carbohydrate" and as carbohydrate stores become depleted during long or intense exercise, fat is not as efficiently used. Finally, fat requires oxygen to be used in exercise. For high-intensity exercise, little fat can be converted into energy as the body is predominantly using carbohydrates in anaerobic metabolism. One of the benefits of cardiovascular exercise training is that it improves the body's ability to use fat as a fuel earlier in an exercise session and at higher intensity levels.

VITAMINS AND MINERALS

Vitamins and minerals are food components that serve essential functions for health. While vitamins and minerals do not directly make energy, they are critical components for energy production. See pages 29 and 30 for a description of all the vitamins and minerals and their roles in health. Three groups of vitamins and minerals that are especially important for active people are discussed in this section.

Electrolytes

Electrolytes include sodium and potassium. These minerals help in maintaining the balance of fluids and are essential in muscle contraction and nerve impulse transmission. Sweating increases not only water loss, but also electrolyte loss. In fact, on average, 1 gram of sodium is lost with every 1 to 2 pounds of sweat.

For exercise lasting longer than 90 minutes, replacing electrolytes is an important consideration. Sports drinks are an easy and convenient way to take in electrolytes during and after exercise. Most people do not have any trouble meeting their sodium requirements from whole foods. Sodium is a component of almost every food we eat, and is present in very high amounts in processed foods. Potassium is a different story; many people do not meet their potassium needs (Table 3.14).

Table 3.14 Potassium in Food

Recommended Intake is 3,500 mg Each Day		
	Serving Size	Amount of Potassium (mg)
Baked potato with skin	1 medium	844
Florida avocado	1/2 medium	742
California avocado	1/2 medium	549
Dried figs	5 each	666
Raisins	1/4 cup	563
Kidney beans	1/2 cup cooked	357
Orange juice	1 cup	474
Spinach	1/2 cup cooked	419
Cantaloupe	1 cup pieces	494

Source: U.S. Department of Agriculture

Antioxidants

Exercise increases the production of compounds called free radicals, which are highly unstable compounds that potentially harm healthy cells, increasing the risk of diseases such as cancer and heart disease. Antioxidant nutrients, nutrients that stabilize the free radicals before they can do any damage, should be included in all diets, especially those of active individuals. While there is no conclusive data on antioxidant nutrient requirements for active people and athletes, many experts agree that athletes have a higher need for these nutrients, especially vitamins C, E, and A (including beta-carotene) (Table 3.15).

Table 3.15 Antioxidants

			Recommendations	
Antioxidant	Athletes	Daily Value (RDA)	US Olympic Committee Guidelines	Upper Limit for Safety
Vitamin E (IU)	400–800	22	100–400	1500
Vitamin C	500–1000	60	250–1000	2000
Vitamin A (IU)		5000		10,000

Source: U.S. Department of Agriculture   Note: IU=International Units

If choosing to take supplements to meet antioxidant requirements, keep in mind that there are upper intake limits for safety. Supplementing with a large amount of beta-carotene can actually increase the risk for lung cancer for people at high risk. So more is not necessarily better in the case of antioxidants. Ensure that needs are met, but do not overdo the supplements. Taking into account the intense activity and extreme environments of fire fighters, a good recommendation for antioxidant intake is 100 to 400 International Units (IU) of vitamin E and 250 to 500 mg of Vitamin C.

B Vitamins

The B vitamins play a critical role in energy production. Athletes with insufficient B-vitamin intake fatigue faster and have a higher lactic acid output when working at lower intensities. Therefore, many sports nutritionists recommend B vitamin intake at two times the RDA for active adults.

Inadequate intake of the B vitamins contributes to the build-up of a toxin that has been implicated as contributing to almost 10% of heart disease deaths. There are many foods that provide B vitamins, yet most American adults do not meet recommended intakes. B vitamins, like other vitamins, can be toxic in large amounts. There is an upper limit for safety for many B vitamins.

Food intake data indicate that male athletes generally meet their nutritional requirements, while the diets of female athletes tend to be deficient in iron, calcium, and zinc.

WATER/FLUIDS

Hydration is critical for optimal performance. Progressive dehydration from exercise impairs performance, and can be life-threatening. It is essential that athletes are well hydrated before and during exercise. For more information about hydration, see page 94.

FOOD INTAKE BEFORE, DURING, AND AFTER EXERCISE

What and when you eat are important considerations for athletes. The goal of nutrition is to minimize fatigue and maximize performance. Nutrition can play a critical role in training and competition by delaying the onset of fatigue during exercise and minimizing post-exercise soreness and recovery time.

Pre-exercise

The purpose of fueling before exercise is to "top off" muscle glycogen (carbohydrate) stores to supply energy to the muscles. As previously described, carbohydrate is the primary fuel for the muscles during intense exercise, and therefore should be the dominant nutrient eaten before competition or training. The pre-competition meal should be easily digestible, high in complex carbohydrates (e.g., bread, pasta, potato), moderate in protein, and low in fat, eaten about three hours before the event. Approximately 1 to 4 grams of carbohydrate per kg of body weight is appropriate for high-intensity exercise. For a 185-pound person, that would be a range of 84 to 336 grams of carbohydrate in the pre-exercise meal. Timing is important. Many people cannot tolerate food right before exercise. Within an hour before competition, consume foods that will digest easily and empty into the bloodstream quickly, such as a bagel, banana, or sport drink.

During Exercise

The nutritional goals during exercise are to keep hydrated, spare muscle glycogen stores, and to maintain electrolyte balance. For "ultra" endurance events, protein in small amounts (10 grams/hour) should be consumed. As a reminder, consume 6 to 12 ounces of fluid every 15 to 20 min when exercising less than an hour; consume 6 to 12 ounces of a 6 to 8% carbohydrate beverage with sodium every 15 to 20 minutes of exercising when exercising for over an hour.

Post-exercise

Muscles utilize significant quantities of energy for contraction. The replenishment of energy stores must come from nutrients within the body. While sore muscles are a sign of a hard workout, they may also be a sign that the fire fighter's post-exercise nutrition is lacking vital ingredients for optimum muscle recovery. During high-intensity exercise, most of the energy comes from muscle carbohydrate (glycogen) energy stores. As muscles use up glycogen stores, energy from amino acids is used. After exercise, successful recovery includes replacing carbohydrate (glycogen) stores and protein for muscle tissue repair.

Muscle recovery is an umbrella term used to describe the physiological processes that occur after exercise to return the body to normal. Rehydration, replenishment of nutrient stores, and reduction of muscle damage and fatigue are essential to muscle recovery. Generally, this process takes between 24 and 48 hours.

There are three phases in post-exercise recovery. First, during the "rapid" phase (0 to 30 min after exercise), the body returns to its normal, pre-exercise state. Lactic acid is removed from muscles and body temperature returns to normal. Replacing body water lost during exercise is the most important nutritional consideration during this time. With as little as a 2% body water shortage, the ability to perform a high-intensity activity can be impaired by up to 35%. Translated into performance, that means a greatly reduced workout or an additional 10 to 20 seconds on skills course time. Water is the key ingredient for rehydration, and sports beverages provide carbohydrates and electrolytes to help recover after exercise.

The second phase in post-exercise muscle recovery is the "intermediate" phase (30 min to 1-1/2 hours after exercise). During the intermediate recovery phase, it is critical to replenish muscle carbohydrate (glycogen) stores and make protein available for making and repairing muscle tissue. Timing is everything; in the hour immediately after exercise the body is most responsive to nutrition replacement. Consuming carbohydrates within an hour after exercise almost doubles the rate of muscle glycogen stores replacement, resulting in more energy for the next workout. Carbohydrate intake is important, and combining carbohydrate with protein promotes the repair and rebuilding of muscle. After exercise, muscle protein building and carbohydrate replenishment is greatest when both protein and carbohydrate are consumed within 30 minutes after exercise.

The bottom line: Consuming 50 to 100 grams of carbohydrate and 10 to 40 grams of protein immediately after exercise replaces depleted muscle energy (glycogen) stores while stimulating muscle building. The end result is reduced muscle fatigue and soreness. Refer to the following examples for recovery food suggestions ranging from 200 to 400 calories that include both protein and carbohydrate:

- 1 oz cereal with 1/2 c milk and a sliced banana
- 1 cup yogurt with sliced fruit
- low-fat soup with whole grain bread
- low fat muffin with a cup of milk
- 1 cup fruit with a bagel filled with sliced meat or low-fat cheese

Nutritional supplements (sports supplements) are not necessary to achieve muscle recovery, but are simply a convenient alternative as long as protein content is not excessive. Too much protein within two hours of exercise can slow fluid and electrolyte replacement.

Finally, the "long-term" phase of exercise muscle recovery is the 2 to 20 hours after exercise. The nutrition goal of the long term post-exercise recovery phase is to ensure that enough total energy (calories) is available to rebuild muscle after exercise, and that enough protein and carbohydrates are available to continue the recovery process started in the intermediate phase. Individual weight and specific physical activities determine recommendations for long-term recovery diets. In general, carbohydrates should be the foundation (>50 to 60% of total food intake), with 1.2 to 2 grams of protein per kg of body weight.

In summary, cover the following key points when working with fire fighters for optimal nutrition:

- Muscle recovery is the physiological process that occurs after exercise to bring the body back to normal. Post-exercise nutrition can shorten muscle recovery time, resulting in improved physical gain from exercise.

- In the rapid muscle recovery phase, rehydrating is the primary nutritional goal.

- During the intermediate recovery phase (up to 1-1/2 hours after exercise), the body is most sensitive to nutrition replacement. A snack of proteins and carbohydrates should be consumed during this period to replace energy stores and hasten the post-exercise muscle building and repair.

- In the long-term recovery phase, diets must include sufficient total calories, as well as adequate protein and carbohydrates to continue the muscle repair and building processes started in the intermediate recovery phase.

BALANCE

Nutrient balance is essential to the active adult for good health. The Food Guide Pyramid shows all the food groups necessary for health and performance. Recommendations for an active individual's diet are shown in Table 3.16.

ERGOGENIC AIDS

It is estimated that almost one half of all Americans take a nutritional supplement of some type. In the athletic population, the percentage who take supplements is even higher. Nutritional supplements used to enhance performance are called ergogenic aids, a term that refers to an increased ability to do work. The nutritional supplement industry is a multi-billion dollar industry in the United States, though it is not closely regulated. This accounts for some of the outrageous claims made by supplement manufacturers. When deciding whether or not to use a nutritional supplement, an individual must keep an open mind and ask questions.

Table 3.17 provides a summary of some the more popular ergogenic aids on the market today. A good resource for more in-depth information is in *The Ergogenics Edge* by Dr. Melvin H. Williams, Human Kinetics Publishers, 1998.

Table 3.16
A general model for food and energy intake for active individuals of different body weights, including a sample 2500 kcal menu containing 350 g of carbohydrate

BODY WEIGHT	110 lb (50 kg)	132 lb (60 kg)	154 lb (70 kg)	176 lb (80 kg)
Total kcal	2500	3000	3500	4000
RECOMMENDED NUMBER OF DAILY SERVINGS				
Milk group (90 kcal) Skim milk 1 cup Plain, low-fat yogurt, 1 cup	4	4	4	4
Meat group (55–75 kcal) Cooked, lean meat (fish, poultry), 1 oz Egg, 1 Peanut butter, 1tbsp Low-fat cheese, 1 oz Cottage cheese, 1/4 cup	5	5	6	6
Fruits	7	9	10	12
Vegetables	3	5	6	7
Grains	16	18	20	24
Lipids	5	6	8	10

SAMPLE HIGH-CARBOHYDRATE 2500-kcal MENU (350 g)

Breakfast	Lunch	Dinner	Snack # 1	Snack #2
1 cup bran cereal	3 oz lean roast beef	Chicken stir-fry:	3 cups popcorn	8 oz apple cider
8 oz low-fat milk	1 hard roll	3 oz chicken		
1 english muffin	2 tsp mayonnaise,	1 cup diced vegetables		
1 tsp margarine	mustard, lettuce,	2 tsp oil		
4 oz orange juice	and tomato	2 cups rice		
	1/2 cup cole slaw	1 cup orange and		
	2 fresh plums	grapefruit sections		
	2 oatmeal cookies	1 cup vanilla yogurt		
	8 oz seltzer water	Iced tea with lemon		
	with lemon			

Source: McArdle, W.D., Katch, F.I., & Katch, V.L. (2000). Essentials of Exercise Physiology, 2/e. Philadephia: Lippincott, Williams & Wilkins.

Table 3.17
Popular Ergogenic Supplements

Ergogenic aid	How it is used in the body	Possible performance benefit (strength of evidence)	Dose	Side Effects
BCAA – Branched Chain Amino Acids (Leucine, Isoleucine, & Valine)	These amino acids are used for fuel during prolonged exercise and provide amino acids for protein synthesis.	May prevent mental fatigue (weak) and muscle protein breakdown (moderate) during prolonged exercise. May assist muscle growth with strength training (weak).	5–20 g/day	May cause gastrointestinal distress at high doses
Caffeine	Stimulates the CNS, the release of epinephrine, free fatty acid mobilization, and the release of calcium in the muscle cell.	May improve endurance (strong) due to glycogen sparing. Increased alertness may improve performance for explosive activities (weak).	5–9 mg/kg of body weight	May cause heart palpitations, nervousness, trembling
Carnitine (L-Carnitine)	Assembled from amino acids in the body. A cofactor for several enzymes in the muscle.	May improve endurance (weak) due to glycogen sparing. May improve $\dot{V}O_2$ max (weak).	.5–.6 g/day	May cause diarrhea at high doses. May interfere with normal L-carnitine functions in the body
Chromium (chromium picolinate, chromium nicotinate)	An essential mineral that works to enhance insulin sensitivity.	May increase muscle mass (weak) and decrease body fat (weak).	200–400 mcg/day	High levels over time may lead to DNA damage
Coenzyme Q10 (CoQ10, Ubiquinone)	Found in the mitochondria. Functions in electron transport system and as an antioxidant.	May improve aerobic exercise performance (research suggests it may hinder performance).	100–150 mg/day	High doses may cause excessive muscle damage during exercise
DHEA (dehydro-epiandrosterone)	Hormone produced by the adrenal gland. Function unknown – may be converted into other hormones.	May decrease body fat (weak) and increase muscle mass (weak).	50–100 mg/day	High doses over time may cause liver damage and prostate cancer
Ephedrine	Stimulates the SNS.	May improve aerobic (weak) and anaerobic (weak) exercise performance.	20–25 mg	May cause nervousness, headache, gastrointestinal distress, irregular heartbeats, and stroke
Glutamine	Made in the body and stored in muscle. Accounts for approximately half of the body's amino acid pool.	Minimizes reduction in immune function (strong) and loss of muscle mass (moderate) during prolonged exercise. Increases muscle mass (weak) and decreases body fat (weak).	.2–.6 g/kg body weight	May cause gastrointestinal distress at high doses
Glycerol	Found in dietary fat. Helps the body store more water by unknown mechanism.	May enhance endurance performance (weak) by preventing dehydration and increasing blood volume.	1 g/kg body weight	May cause headaches or nausea
HMB (beta-hydroxy-beta-methylbutyrate)	Byproduct of leucine metabolism. Unknown action in the body.	May increase muscle mass (weak) and decrease body fat (weak).	1.3–3.0 g/day	No reported adverse side effects
Yohimbine	Increases PSNS activity. Possible increases in metabolism and testosterone production.	May increase muscle mass (weak) and decrease body fat (weak).	15–20 mg/day	May produce dizziness, nervousness, headache, nausea, or vomiting

Note: SNS = Sympathetic Nervous System; PSNS = Parasympathetic Nervous System

Adapted from Williams, M.H. (1998). The Ergogenics Edge. *Champaign, Ill.: Human Kinetics.*

CONCLUSION

Success in achieving peak performance is primarily influenced by three factors: genetics, training, and nutrition. While there is not much anyone can do about their heredity, physical training programs and eating habits can be modified. Eating the right foods at the right time can maximize benefits from training and improve physical performance.

Practical Application of Nutrition for PFTs

1. Completion of food log and calculation of daily caloric intake (Table 3.18):
   - ❏ The purpose of a food log is to make the fire fighter aware of the quantity AND the quality of the foods they are consuming.
   - ❏ Have the fire fighter complete a food log for three to five days. At least one of the days should be a weekend day. If the client is a fire fighter, at least one day should be a day on shift.
   - ❏ The food log should include: food description, quantity, calories, fat grams, carb grams, protein grams.
   - ❏ The fire fighter should calculate average daily caloric intake. The fire fighter will need to obtain a food guide for personal use or have access to a simple nutrition analysis program.

2. PFT should calculate recommended daily caloric intake using one of the formulas in this section.

3. Discuss basic nutrition concepts with the fire fighter, for example:
   - ❏ Balancing the Food Guide Pyramid
   - ❏ Decreasing portion sizes
   - ❏ Making healthy food choices
   - ❏ How to read food labels
   - ❏ Proper hydration
   - ❏ Weight loss: Consume 500 calories less, exercise 500+ calories more

4. Give the fire fighter resources to further explore nutrition concepts including names of registered dietitians, nutritionists, Web sites, books, and articles, for example:
   - ❏ http://www.acsm.org/
   - ❏ http://www.ag.uiuc.edu/~food-lab/nat/add_amt.cgi
   - ❏ http://dawp.anet.com/
   - ❏ http://www.cyberdiet.com/
   - ❏ http://www.nat.uiuc.edu/

Table 3.18
Sample Food Log

Date	Time of Day	Qty	Description of Food/Beverage	Calories	Fat/Carbs/ Protein	Protein	Carbs

On back, please list any supplements and/or vitamins you currently use.

REFERENCE:

Williams, M.H. (1998). *The Ergogenics Edge*. Champaign, Ill.: Human Kinetics.

HEALTH SCREENING
AND
ASSESSMENTS

PEER FITNESS TRAINER ASSESSMENT GUIDELINES

BLOOD PRESSURE CLASSIFICATION

Medical screening is required yearly for all uniformed personnel. This screening includes blood pressure measurements to determine the presence or absence of hypertension. Hypertension is a major risk factor for heart disease. Blood pressure classification is based on the average of two or more measurements taken on two or more occasions after initial screening. A normotensive individual can have mildly elevated blood pressure prior to their fitness assessment due to anxiety or other acute stresses. If after a brief rest of five minutes, an individual's blood pressure is within normal limits (under 140/90), the testing may proceed. If blood pressure remains *mildly* elevated (under 160/100), and the individual has been medically cleared within the last year and has no more than two other risk factors listed on page 157 of the *ACE Personal Trainer Manual*, then fitness testing can continue.

Individuals who remain mildly hypertensive and who have two or more other risk factors, or have not been recently medically cleared, should be referred to their personal or departmental physician for medical evaluation.

All individuals who present with moderate hypertension that does not improve with a rest period should not receive fitness assessments and should be referred to their personal or departmental physician.

Peer Fitness Trainers must emphasize the importance of periodic blood pressure monitoring for all individuals, especially those at risk for hypertension, and advise lifestyle modifications where appropriate (Table 4.1 and Figure 4.1). They must also be careful to

CHAPTER

avoid causing disproportionate concern for mild elevations that might be due to temporary anxiety or acute stress. All participants should be advised about the risk factors for hypertension, including heredity, obesity, and cigarette smoking.

Table 4.1		
Blood Pressure Summary for uniformed personnel completing a medical exam within the past 12 months		
Low Risk < 139/89	Moderate Risk 140–159/90–99	High Risk >160/100

Figure 4.1

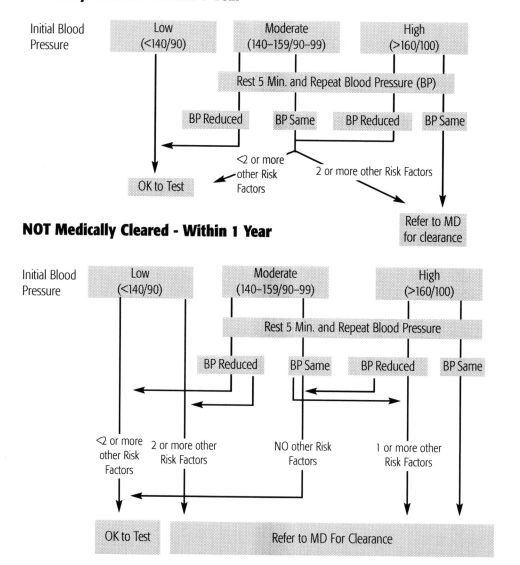

PRE-FITNESS ASSESSMENT BLOOD PRESSURE SCREENING

MUSCULAR STRENGTH TESTING AND CALCULATING TRAINING LOAD

Muscular strength testing is discussed in the ACE Personal Trainer Manual *on pages 197–201.*

One repetition maximum (1RM) testing is used by athletic trainers, physical therapists, and fitness professionals to quantify the level of strength, assess imbalances, and to design and evaluate strength-training programs. Extreme efforts or maximal exertions are not recommended for individuals who are untrained, inexperienced, injured, medically supervised, elderly, cardiac patients, or adolescents. For these populations, and even the fitness client, the 1 RM conversion chart is a safe, effective, and reliable tool (Table 4.2).

When testing a client, strict adherence to proper and safe exercise form is of utmost importance. If performing this test with an inexperienced client, teach the client the proper form using the "Tell-Show-Do" teaching technique discussed in Chapter 14 of the *ACE Personal Trainer Manual*. The client should be able to demonstrate proper form before proceeding with strength testing.

PROTOCOL FOR USING 1 RM CONVERSION CHART

The 1 RM Conversion Chart is based on the following formula:

1RM = weight lifted divided by 1.0278 – [.0278 x (number of reps completed)]

(Brzycki, 1993; National Strength and Conditioning Association, 2000)

The goal of the testing is to determine the heaviest weight that can be lifted for 10 repetitions or less.

Testing Protocol:

1. Instruct the client to warm up for 5 to 8 minutes.

2. If desired, the client may perform some light stretches using the target muscles.

3. The client will perform one warm-up set with light resistance (approximately 50%) for 8 to 12 repetitions.

4. Provide a 1-minute rest.

5. Estimate a conservative, near max load. If the client appears to be able to complete more than 10 reps, stop the bout around 6 to 8 repetitions.

6. Provide a 2- to 3-minute rest.

7. Choose a heavier load and proceed with the testing. Always provide a 2- to 3- minute rest between bouts.

8. Once a weight has been determined to be the amount that can be lifted less than 10 reps, refer to the chart.

9. Find the weight in the left hand column and the number of repetitions on the top line. The point at which the two amounts intersect on the chart is the estimated maximum weight.

Table 4.2 1 Repetition Maximum Conversion Chart

$$1\ RM = \frac{WEIGHT}{1.0278 - .0278(REPS)}$$

REPETITIONS

WT	1	2	3	4	5	6	7	8	9	10
20	20	21	21	22	23	23	24	25	26	27
25	25	26	26	27	28	29	30	31	32	33
30	30	31	32	33	34	35	36	37	39	41
35	35	36	37	38	39	41	42	43	45	47
40	40	41	42	44	45	46	48	50	51	53
45	45	46	48	49	51	52	54	56	58	60
50	50	51	53	55	56	58	60	62	64	67
55	55	57	58	60	62	64	66	68	71	73
60	60	62	64	65	67	70	72	74	77	80
65	65	67	69	71	73	75	78	81	84	87
70	70	72	74	76	79	81	84	87	90	93
75	75	77	79	82	84	87	90	93	96	100
80	80	82	85	87	90	93	96	99	103	107
85	85	87	90	93	96	99	102	106	109	113
90	90	93	95	98	101	105	108	112	116	120
95	95	98	101	104	107	110	114	118	122	127
100	100	103	106	109	112	116	120	124	129	133
105	105	108	111	115	118	122	126	130	135	140
110	110	113	116	120	124	128	132	137	141	147
115	115	118	122	125	129	134	138	143	148	153
120	120	123	127	131	135	139	144	149	154	160
125	125	129	132	136	141	145	150	155	161	167
130	130	134	138	142	146	151	156	161	167	173
135	135	139	143	147	152	157	162	168	174	180
140	140	144	148	153	157	163	168	174	180	187
145	145	149	154	158	164	169	174	180	186	193
150	150	154	159	164	169	174	180	186	193	200
155	155	159	164	169	174	180	186	192	199	207
160	160	165	170	175	180	186	192	199	206	213
165	165	170	175	180	186	192	198	205	212	220
170	170	175	180	185	191	197	204	211	219	227
175	175	180	185	191	197	203	210	217	225	233

REPETITIONS

WT	1	2	3	4	5	6	7	8	9	10
180	180	185	191	196	202	209	216	223	231	240
185	185	190	196	202	208	215	222	230	238	247
190	190	195	201	207	214	221	228	236	244	253
195	195	200	206	213	219	226	234	242	251	260
200	200	205	212	218	225	232	240	248	257	267
205	205	210	217	224	231	238	246	254	264	273
210	210	215	222	229	236	244	252	261	270	280
215	215	220	228	235	242	250	258	267	276	287
220	220	225	233	240	247	255	264	273	283	293
225	225	230	238	245	253	261	270	279	289	300
230	230	235	244	251	259	267	276	286	296	307
235	235	242	249	256	264	273	282	292	302	313
240	240	247	254	262	270	279	288	298	309	320
245	245	252	259	267	276	285	294	304	315	327
250	250	257	265	273	281	290	300	310	321	333
255	255	262	270	278	287	296	306	317	328	340
260	260	267	275	284	292	302	312	323	334	347
265	265	273	281	289	298	308	318	329	341	353
270	270	278	286	295	304	314	324	335	347	360
275	275	283	291	300	309	319	330	341	354	367
280	280	288	296	305	315	325	336	348	360	373
285	285	293	302	311	321	331	342	354	366	380
290	290	298	307	316	326	337	348	360	373	387
295	295	303	312	322	332	343	354	366	379	393
300	300	309	318	327	337	348	360	372	386	400
305	305	314	323	333	343	354	366	379	392	407
310	310	319	328	338	349	360	372	385	399	413
315	315	324	334	344	354	366	378	391	405	420
320	320	329	339	349	360	372	384	397	412	427
325	325	334	344	355	366	377	390	404	418	433
330	330	339	349	360	371	383	396	410	424	440
335	335	345	355	365	377	389	402	416	431	447

Reprinted with permission from the Journal of Physical Education, Recreation & Dance, a publication of the American Alliance for Health, Physical Education, Recreation and Dance, 1900 Association Dr., Reston, VA 2019I.

CALCULATING TRAINING LOAD

The maximum weight lifted is an effective tool to use in calculating loads for programming of strength training. This is discussed in the *ACE Personal Trainer Manual*, Chapters 8 and 9.

LEG PRESS AND BENCH PRESS RATIO

A good way to assess the relative strength of people of different sizes is to make pound-for-pound comparisons. You will find an example of such a comparison on the following pages. These comparisons were established on a universal strength system and therefore are only valid on that system. In addition, the comparisons do not account for other confounding factors such as differences in body composition, muscle fiber type, and training experience. Therefore, as with any table of norms, this should be used only as a guideline (Table 4.3).

Table 4.3   **CHEST PRESS RATIOS**   CHEST PRESS RATIO = $\dfrac{\text{WEIGHT PUSHED}}{\text{BODY WT.}}$

MEN			AGE					WOMEN			AGE			
%	<20	20-29	30-39	40-49	50-59	60+		%	<20	20-29	30-39	40-49	50-59	60+
99	>1.76	>1.63	>1.35	>1.20	>1.05	>.94		99	>.88	>1.01	>.82	>.77	>.68	>.72
95	1.76	1.63	1.35	1.20	1.05	0.94	SUPERIOR	95	0.88	1.01	0.82	0.77	0.68	0.72
90	1.46	1.48	1.24	1.10	0.97	0.89		90	0.83	0.90	0.76	0.71	0.61	0.64
85	1.38	1.37	1.17	1.04	0.93	0.84		85	0.81	0.83	0.72	0.66	0.57	0.59
80	1.34	1.32	1.12	1.00	0.90	0.82	EXCELLENT	80	0.77	0.80	0.70	0.62	0.55	0.54
75	1.29	1.26	1.08	0.96	0.87	0.79		75	0.76	0.77	0.65	0.60	0.53	0.53
70	1.24	1.22	1.04	0.93	0.84	0.77		70	0.74	0.74	0.63	0.57	0.52	0.51
65	1.23	1.18	1.01	0.90	0.81	0.74		65	0.70	0.72	0.62	0.55	0.50	0.48
60	1.19	1.14	0.98	0.88	0.79	0.72	GOOD	60	0.65	0.70	0.60	0.54	0.48	0.47
55	1.16	1.10	0.96	0.86	0.77	0.70		55	0.64	0.68	0.58	0.53	0.47	0.46
50	1.13	1.06	0.93	0.84	0.75	0.68		50	0.63	0.65	0.58	0.52	0.46	0.45
45	1.10	1.03	0.90	0.82	0.73	0.67		45	0.60	0.63	0.55	0.51	0.45	0.44
40	1.06	0.99	0.88	0.80	0.71	0.66	FAIR	40	0.58	0.59	0.53	0.50	0.44	0.43
35	1.01	0.96	0.86	0.78	0.70	0.65		35	0.57	0.58	0.52	0.48	0.43	0.41
30	0.96	0.93	0.83	0.76	0.68	0.63		30	0.56	0.56	0.51	0.47	0.42	0.40
25	0.93	0.90	0.81	0.74	0.66	0.60		25	0.55	0.53	0.49	0.45	0.41	0.39
20	0.89	0.88	0.78	0.72	0.63	0.57	POOR	20	0.53	0.51	0.47	0.43	0.39	0.38
15	0.86	0.84	0.75	0.69	0.60	0.56		15	0.52	0.50	0.45	0.42	0.38	0.36
10	0.81	0.80	0.71	0.65	0.57	0.53		10	0.50	0.48	0.42	0.38	0.37	0.33
5	0.76	0.72	0.65	0.59	0.53	0.49		5	0.41	0.44	0.39	0.35	0.31	0.26
1	<.76	<.72	<.65	<.59	<.53	<.49		1	<.41	<.436	<.39	<.35	<.305	<.26

Source: The Physical Fitness Specialist Manual, *The Cooper Institute, Dallas, Texas, revised 2002, reprinted with permission.*

FITNESS PROTOCOLS

Fitness protocols are used to determine the uniformed personnel's baseline level of fitness and to evaluate progress from year to year. Fitness evaluations shall be under the auspices of the fire department physician. The actual evaluations may be conducted by the fire department's fitness personnel. All data collected by the evaluator are to be held confidential and maintained in the uniformed personnel's confidential medical file. The evaluator may provide exercise programs to encourage the uniformed personnel to maintain or improve their level of fitness.

> The fitness protocols have been extensively revised since the original release of the Wellness-Fitness Initiative. The revisions of all maintained protocols, and the deletion of others, were done to accurately evaluate uniformed personnel fitness levels and decrease errors in data collection. Use of earlier protocols and equipment or substitution of other protocols and equipment is not allowed.

There are many protocols currently available to measure the sub-maximal $\dot{V}O_2$ levels of apparently healthy individuals. These protocols differ in evaluation equipment (i.e., treadmill, stairmill, step, and stationary bike), rate of increasing work output, degree of increasing work output, and final result. To increase the consistency of $\dot{V}O_2$ measurements, as well as the accuracy of the data collected between uniformed personnel within and between participating fire departments, two sub-maximal protocols are being maintained for measuring aerobic capacity. These are the Gerkin Treadmill Protocol and the FDNY Stairmill Protocol. Both protocols were specifically developed and validated to evaluate the sub-maximal aerobic capacity of uniformed personnel.

After continued evaluation and research by the Wellness-Fitness Initiative's technical experts, it was determined that significant errors were occurring when past protocols were applied to a population that has different characteristics from those for which the evaluation was developed. For this reason, the Bruce and Balke Treadmill Protocols were removed as evaluation protocols and as a means to collect data. Both Bruce and Balke were specifically tailored for less fit populations to determine cardiovascular pathology and thus proved to be less accurate protocols for the general uniformed personnel population. The YMCA Stationary Bike Test Protocol was also removed since it consistently and grossly underestimated $\dot{V}O_2$ for above average body size (i.e., most uniformed personnel). The Canadian Step Test was also removed from the Wellness-Fitness Initiative since it relies on a single stage exercise that was found to underestimate measurement of uniformed personnel's $\dot{V}O_2$.

A maximal cardiopulmonary evaluation with an electrocardiogram (ECG) can also be used to obtain $\dot{V}O_2$ measurements. This medical evaluation shall only be conducted in a medical facility with proper monitoring by a physician and available resuscitation equipment.

The muscular endurance evaluations were also modified. In order to improve the accuracy of the evaluation and the data collection, the sit and hold evaluation was eliminated. The sit-up protocol was changed to a curl-up evaluation in order to ensure the safety of the participant and to improve the specificity of the evaluation. The push-up evaluation was modified to ensure uniformity in data collection.

The flexibility evaluation was modified to address the difference in limb length and/or differences in proportion between an individual's arm and legs.

EVALUATION EQUIPMENT

All evaluation equipment must be obtained and used as specified in these protocols. The Wellness-Fitness Initiative's technical experts have evaluated all equipment utilized in the original protocols. The technical experts found either accuracy, maintenance, or availability problems with some evaluation equipment. Accordingly, equipment changes have been made from the original manual. Manufacturer's information, product names, and model numbers are included in each protocol. Unless indicated, this equipment must not be substituted with other equipment. All equipment must be maintained and properly calibrated in accordance with the manufacturer's instructions.

The following fitness evaluations with the corresponding protocols and equipment are to be used for the Wellness-Fitness Initiative:

AEROBIC CAPACITY

- Treadmill – Submaximal treadmill evaluations shall use the Gerkin Treadmill Protocol. The treadmill shall be a LifeFitness 9100HR or a commercial treadmill capable of obtaining a 15% grade and 10 mph. The fire department must verify that the treadmill is equivalent to the LifeFitness 9100HR. A Polar Heart Rate Monitor shall be used for heart rate measurements and a stopwatch used for timing.

- Stairmill – Submaximal stairmill evaluations shall use the FDNY Stairmill Protocol. The stairmill shall be a StairMaster 7000PT. A Polar Heart Rate Monitor shall be used for heart rate measurements and a stopwatch used for timing.

- Treadmill – Maximal treadmill evaluations shall use a continuous, multigrade medical cardiovascular protocol utilizing a electrocardiogram (ECG) for cardiac measurements. This evaluation must be under the direct supervision of a physician. The treadmill shall be a commercial treadmill capable of obtaining a 25% grade.

MUSCULAR STRENGTH

- Hand Grip Dynamometer – Hand grip strength evaluations shall use the Wellness-Fitness Initiative Protocol for Hand Grip. The hand grip dynamometer shall be a Jamar Hydraulic Hand dynamometer.

- Arm Dynamometer – Arm strength evaluations shall use the Wellness-Fitness Initiative Protocol for Arm Strength. The arm dynamometer shall be the Jackson Strength

Evaluation System or a commercial dynamometer system that is digital, incorporates dead load cells, and includes an adjustable chain, handle bar, and test platform. The fire department must verify that the dynamometer is equivalent to the Jackson Strength Evaluation System. A straight-grip handlebar is required.

- Leg Dynamometer — Leg strength evaluations shall use the Wellness-Fitness Initiative Protocol for Leg Strength. The leg dynamometer shall be the Jackson Strength Evaluation System or a commercial dynamometer system that is digital, incorporates dead load cells, and includes an adjustable chain, handle bar, and test platform. The fire department must verify that the dynamometer is equivalent to the Jackson Strength Evaluation System. A V-grip handlebar (chinning triangle) is required.

MUSCULAR ENDURANCE

- Push-up — Push-up muscle endurance evaluations shall use the Wellness-Fitness Initiative Protocol for Push-ups. Equipment used for this evaluation include a five-inch prop (i.e., cup, sponge), a metronome, and a stopwatch.

- Curl-up — Curl-up muscle endurance evaluations shall use the Wellness-Fitness Initiative Protocol for Curl-ups. Equipment used for this evaluation include a gym mat, a metronome, and a stopwatch.

FLEXIBILITY

- Sit and Reach — Sit and reach flexibility evaluations shall use the Wellness-Fitness Initiative Sit and Reach Protocol. Equipment used for this evaluation shall be a Novel Acuflex I or equivalent trunk flexibility tester that compensates for variable arm and leg lengths.

EVALUATION SEQUENCE

Uniformed personnel must be fully recovered from the previous evaluation before proceeding to the next evaluation. The evaluation events may be sequenced to minimize the effects of previous evaluations on subsequent evaluation performance. If evaluations for aerobic capacity, muscular strength, muscle endurance, and flexibility are to be evaluated in one evaluation battery, the following sequence should be used:

1. Resting heart rate and resting blood pressure

2. Aerobic capacity

3. Muscle strength

4. Muscle endurance

5. Flexibility

MANDATORY PRE-EVALUATION PROCEDURE

The following is a mandatory pre-evaluation procedure. It shall be conducted for all uniformed personnel prior to conducting the fitness evaluations:

- Review and confirm individual's current medical status. **It is required that all uniformed personnel are medically cleared through the Wellness-Fitness Initiative's medical evaluation within 12 months prior to any fitness evaluation.**

- Notify uniformed personnel in advance of the scheduled time and place of physical fitness evaluations. The individual should understand the protocol and what is expected before, during, and after the evaluation, including start and stop procedures. Individual will be required to wear comfortable clothes and either sneakers or athletic shoes. All uniformed personnel must refrain from eating, drinking, smoking, and any physical activity prior to the evaluation to ensure accurate heart rate and blood pressure measurements.

- Obtain a resting heart rate and blood pressure prior to aerobic capacity evaluation. If resting heart rate exceeds 110 beats per minute and/or resting blood pressure exceeds 160/100 mm Hg, ask the individual to relax in a quiet place for five minutes and re-test. If the heart rate and/or blood pressure remain at these levels, cancel the fitness evaluation and refer the individual to the fire department physician. If the re-test indicates a reduction in heart rate and blood pressure, the evaluation may be given. The aerobic capacity protocols also require that age (both protocols) and weight in kilograms (FDNY protocol only) be obtained prior to the evaluation.

- Review health status with the individual being evaluated. Contraindications for evaluations shall be reviewed, addressing any changes in the individual's health status since his or her last medical evaluation that would warrant deferring the evaluation, including:

  - Unexplained chest pain;

  - Loss of consciousness;

  - Loss of balance due to dizziness (ataxia);

  - Recent injury resulting in bone, joint, or muscle problem;

  - Current prescribed drug that inhibits physical activity;

  - Chronic infectious disease (e.g., hepatitis);

  - Pregnancy;

  - Any recent disorders that may be exacerbated by exercise;

  - Any other reason why the individual believes that he or she should not be physically evaluated

INDICATIONS FOR STOPPING EVALUATION

For all fitness evaluations, the following must be adhered to for premature cessation of the evaluation:

1. Onset of angina or angina-like symptoms.

2. Signs of poor perfusion: light-headedness, confusion, ataxia, pallor, cyanosis, nausea, or cold clammy skin.

3. Failure of heart rate to increase with increase in exercise intensity.

4. Individual requests evaluation to stop.

5. Physical or verbal manifestations of severe fatigue.

6. Failure of the testing equipment.

AEROBIC CAPACITY EVALUATIONS

Aerobic Capacity – The Wellness-Fitness Initiative provides two protocols to determine a fire fighter's sub-maximal aerobic capacity: the Gerkin sub-maximal treadmill protocol and the FDNY sub-maximal stairmill protocol. Through the calculations provided in the respective section, both protocols can successfully estimate a fire fighter's maximal aerobic capacity, which is expressed as $\dot{V}O_2$max. Either of these two protocols can be used by the fire departments that adopt the Wellness-Fitness Initiative, as long as the same evaluation is consistently used for all uniformed personnel within that department and the collected data are specifically attributed to the utilized protocol. Results of aerobic capacity over time must be compared to the same protocol. If the fire department changes protocols, a new baseline $\dot{V}O_2$max must be established. All aerobic capacity evaluation results must be recorded in milligrams of oxygen per kilograms of body weight per minute ($\dot{V}O_2$max).

PRE-EVALUATION PROCEDURES

- Choose the aerobic capacity protocol and worksheet.

- Inform the fire fighter of all evaluation components. Ensure that the individual is in proper clothing and footwear, is comfortable, and understands all facets of the evaluation.

- Review all indicators for stopping the evaluation with the individual.

- Place and secure heart rate monitor transmitter around the individual's chest, in accordance with the manufacturer's instructions. Evaluator shall hold or wear the heart rate monitor wrist receiver.

- Measure the fire fighter's resting heart rate and resting blood pressure and record on the protocol worksheet.

- Obtain and record weight (for FDNY protocol only) and age (for both protocols).

- Determine 85% of the fire fighter's estimated maximum heart rate, which will be the target exercise heart rate, using the following simple percent of heart rate maximum equation:

  Target exercise heart rate = .85 (220 − age)

  Example: The target exercise heart rate of a 40-year-old individual is:
  Target exercise heart rate = .85 (220 − 40) = 153

- Record the target exercise heart rate on the protocol worksheet.

TREADMILL EVALUATION

Submaximal Graded Treadmill Evaluation (Gerkin Protocol)

Equipment

LifeFitness 9100HR or verified equivalent commercial treadmill
Polar Heart Rate Monitor
Stopwatch

Protocol

1. Conduct Pre-Evaluation Procedures.

2. The individual being evaluated is instructed to straddle the treadmill belt until it begins to move. At approximately one mph, the individual is instructed to step onto the belt and the belt speed is increased to three mph at 0% grade. The individual warms up at three mph at 0% grade for three minutes. During the warm-up, the individual is informed that the evaluation is submaximal and will terminate once their monitored heart rate exceeds the target exercise heart rate for 15 seconds. The individual is informed that the target exercise heart rate is 85% of their predicted maximal heart rate. The individual is advised that the evaluation is a series of one-minute exercise stages, alternating between percent grade and speed (i.e., first minute percent grade is increased, second minute speed is increased, etc.). Inform the individual that if at anytime during the evaluation they experience chest pain, light-headedness, ataxia, confusion, nausea, or clamminess, they should ask the evaluator to terminate the evaluation.

3. The individual is informed that the belt speed will gradually increase to the starting speed of 4.5 mph and 0% grade, at which Stage I begins. The individual is permitted to either walk or run, whichever feels more comfortable.

4. During the evaluation, the individual's heart rate is continuously monitored and the heart rate is recorded during the last quarter (15 seconds) of each stage. At the completion of the first minute (stage 1: 4.5 mph @ 0% grade), the grade should be increased to 2%. Subsequently, after every odd minute the grade will be increased an additional 2%. After every even minute the speed will be increased 0.5 mph. This will continue until the individual's heart rate exceeds their target exercise heart rate or demonstrates any of the criteria for early termination of the treadmill evaluation.

5. Once the individual's heart rate exceeds the target exercise heart rate, the individual continues the evaluation for an additional 15 seconds. This 15-second period allows for the individual's heart rate to stabilize. During this stabilization period, the evaluation will remain at the stage where the target exercise heart rate is exceeded, with speed or grade unchanged. If the heart rate does not return to or below the target exercise heart rate the evaluation ends and the final evaluation stage will be recorded.

6. If the evaluation is terminated early, the stage at which the evaluation is terminated and the reason for the termination is documented. For data collection, record that the evaluation was terminated.

7. Once the individual exceeds their target exercise heart rate or reaches the eleventh minute of the evaluation, the evaluation is ended and the final stage is recorded.

8. The individual is instructed to remain on the treadmill for a cool-down period for a minimum of three minutes at three mph, 0% grade. Continue to monitor the heart rate during the cool-down period. Record the heart rate after one minute of cooldown.

9. Use the final stage and the conversion table at right to establish $\dot{V}O_2$max.

10. Record the $\dot{V}O_2$max.

Source: Richard Gerkin, MD, Director of Health Center, Phoenix Fire Department.

SUBMAXIMAL TREADMILL EVALUATION CONVERSION TABLE

STAGE	TIME	CONVERTED $\dot{V}O_2$max
1	1:00	31.15
2.1	1:15	32.55
2.2	1:30	33.6
2.3	1:45	34.65
2.4	2:00	35.35
3.1	2:15	37.45
3.2	2:30	39.55
3.3	2:45	41.30
3.4	3:00	43.4
4.1	3:15	44.1
4.2	3:30	45.15
4.3	3:45	46.2
4.4	4:00	46.5
5.1	4:15	48.6
5.2	4:30	50
5.3	4:45	51.4
5.4	5:00	52.8
6.1	5:15	53.9
6.2	5:30	54.9
6.3	5:45	56
6.4	6:00	57
7.1	6:15	57.7
7.2	6:30	58.8
7.3	6:45	60.2
7.4	7:00	61.2
8.1	7:15	62.3
8.2	7:30	63.3
8.3	7:45	64
8.4	8:00	65
9.1	8:15	66.5
9.2	8:30	68.2
9.3	8:45	69
9.4	9:00	70.7
10.1	9:15	72.1
10.2	9:30	73.1
10.3	9:45	73.8
10.4	10:00	74.9
11.1	10:15	76.3
11.2	10:30	77.7
11.3	10:45	79.1
11.4	11:00	80

STAIRMILL EVALUATION

Submaximal Stepmill Evaluation (FDNY Protocol)

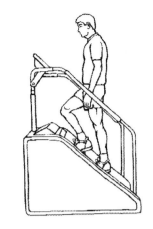

Equipment

StairMaster 7000 PT Stepmill
Polar Heart Rate Monitor
Stopwatch

Protocol

1. Conduct Pre-Evaluation Procedures.
    Obtain and record individual's age in years
    and weight (males only) in kilograms.

2. The individual being evaluated is instructed to assume a starting position about two-thirds of the way up the stairs. The individual is instructed to temporarily grasp the handrails to reduce the possibility of losing balance when the stairs begin to move. The individual is also informed that holding or leaning on the handrails is not allowed once the evaluation begins since this will cause false overestimations of aerobic capacity.

3. The evaluation will commence at Level 3 for a 30-second warm-up period. During this time, the individual is instructed to remove both hands from the handrail, establish a steady rhythm, and walk with their hands by their sides. The individual is informed that the evaluation is submaximal and will terminate in three minutes. The individual is advised that if at anytime during the evaluation they experience chest pain, light-headedness, ataxia, confusion, nausea, or clamminess, they should ask the evaluator to terminate the evaluation.

4. If the evaluation is terminated early, the time at which the evaluation terminated and the reason for the termination is documented. For data collection, record that the evaluation was terminated.

5. At the conclusion of the warm-up the stairmill will be set to Level 4, which begins the actual evaluation time. The individual will walk at a constant rate of 60 steps per minute for three minutes. Heart rate is measured during the final 15 seconds of the exercise and recorded.

6. Upon completion of the evaluation, the individual is instructed to re-grasp the handrails, the stepping machine is shut off, and the individual is assisted off the apparatus.

7. The following equations are used to establish $\dot{V}O_2max$:

    Male $\dot{V}O_2max$ = 113.34 − .15 (weight) − .32 (final heart rate) − .54 (age)
    Female $\dot{V}O_2max$ = 88.22 − .31 (final heart rate) − .32 (age)

8. Record the $\dot{V}O_2max$.

    NOTE: This protocol has been validated as accurate when final heart rate equals or is greater than 110 bpm.

GRIP STRENGTH

Wellness-Fitness Initiative Handgrip Muscle Strength Evaluation Protocol

Equipment

Jamar Hydraulic Hand dynamometer
Towel

Protocol

1. Conduct Pre-Evaluation Procedures.

2. The individual being evaluated is instructed to towel hands to ensure they are dry. The individual is instructed to place the dynamometer in the hand to be evaluated; the evaluator adjusts, ensuring that the bottom of the handle clip is adjusted to fit snug in the first proximal interphalangeal joint. The red peak-hold needle is rotated counterclockwise to the "0" position. The individual is advised that the evaluation is a series of six measurements — three for each hand. The individual is informed that the isometric contraction (squeezing) required during this evaluation must be eased into and then released slowly, without swinging arm, pumping arm, or jerking hand. Inform the individual that if at any time during the evaluation they experience chest pain, light-headedness, ataxia, confusion, nausea, or clamminess, they should terminate the evaluation.

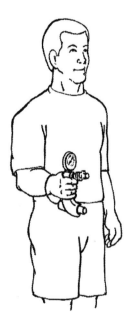

3. The individual is instructed to assume a slightly bent forward position, with elbow bent at a 90-degree angle, shoulder adducted and neutrally rotated, forearm and wrist in neutral position.

4. The individual is instructed to squeeze with maximum strength for two to three seconds while exhaling and then slowly release grip. The peak-hold needle will automatically record the highest force exerted.

5. Measure both hands alternatively allowing three evaluations per hand. Reset the peak-hold needle to zero before obtaining new readings. List the scores for each hand to the nearest kilogram.

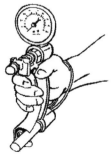

6. Record the highest score.

LEG STRENGTH

Wellness-Fitness Initiative Leg Muscle Strength Evaluation Protocol

Equipment

Jackson Strength Evaluation System with V-Grip Handlebar (chinning triangle) *or*
Verified equivalent dynamometer with V-Grip Handlebar (chinning triangle)
Towel

Protocol

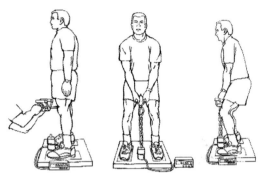

1. Conduct Pre-Evaluation Procedures.

2. The individual being evaluated is instructed to towel hands to ensure they are dry. The individual is advised that the evaluation is a series of three measurements. The individual is informed that the isometric leg extension required during this evaluation must be eased into and then released slowly, without bending back, swinging arm, pumping or bending arm, or jerking hand. Inform the individual that if at any time during the evaluation they experience back pain, chest pain, light-headedness, ataxia, confusion, nausea, or clamminess, they should terminate the evaluation.

3. The individual is instructed to stand upon the dynamometer base plate, which has been placed on a level and secure surface, with feet spread shoulder-width apart. The individual is instructed to stand erect. The chain is then adjusted so the upper (inside) edge of the bottom cross member of the V-grip handlebar is at the top of the individual's knee cap. The evaluator verifies this position, ensuring the chain is taut.

4. The individual is then instructed to hold the bar, look straight with head in the neutral position, fully extend arms, and maintain a straight back. The evaluator shall verify this position and ensure that the individual's hips are directly over their feet, with trunk and knees slightly bent.

5. Instruct the individual to lift using their legs for a total of three seconds.

6. After three seconds, instruct the individual to slowly relax the arms and legs, and to remain at standing rest for 30 seconds.

7. Once the individual has completed the 30-second recovery period, begin the second evaluation. Repeat the evaluation for the third time using the same procedure.

8. List all scores. *Note: Digital readout will display the actual force, the highest peak force, and the average force achieved during the three evaluations.*

9. Record the highest of the three trials to the nearest kilogram.

ARM STRENGTH

Wellness-Fitness Initiative Arm Muscle Strength Evaluation Protocol

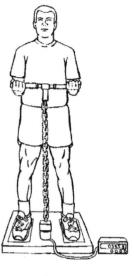

Equipment

Jackson Strength Evaluation System with Straight Handlebar *or*
Verified equivalent dynamometer with Straight Handlebar
Towel

Protocol

1. Conduct Pre-Evaluation Procedures.

2. The individual being evaluated is instructed to towel hands to ensure they are dry. The individual is advised that the evaluation is a series of three measurements. The individual is informed that the isometric arm contraction required during this evaluation must be eased into and then released slowly, without swinging arm, pumping arm, or jerking hands. Inform the individual that if at anytime during the evaluation they experience back pain, chest pain, light-headedness, ataxia, confusion, nausea, or clamminess, they should terminate the evaluation.

3. The individual is instructed to stand upon the dynamometer base plate, which has been placed on a level and secure surface, with feet spread shoulder-width apart. The individual is instructed to hold the bar with a wide grip and bend their elbows 90 degrees (keeping their elbows to their sides). Individual must stand erect without arching back.

4. The instructor verifies that the arm/elbow joint angle is 90 degrees and adjusts the chain so that it is taut in this position.

5. The individual shall be instructed not to shrug shoulders, bend back, or perform any motion other than to contract arms and attempt to move the handlebar in a vertical direction.

6. Instruct the individual to flex arms for a total of three seconds.

7. After three seconds, instruct the individual to slowly relax arms, and to remain at standing rest for 30 seconds.

8. Once the individual has completed the 30-second recovery period, begin the second evaluation. Repeat evaluation for the third time using the same procedure.

9. List all scores. *Note: Digital readout will display the actual force, the highest peak force and the average force achieved during the three evaluations.*

10. Record the highest of the three trials to the nearest kilogram.

PUSH-UP

Wellness-Fitness Initiative Push-up Evaluation Protocol

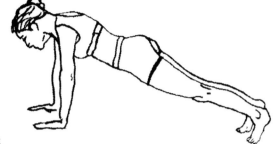

Equipment

Five-inch prop (i.e., cup; sponge)
Metronome
Stopwatch

Protocol

1. Conduct Pre-Evaluation Procedures.

2. The individual is advised that the evaluation is a series of push-ups performed in a two-minute time period. The individual is advised that the evaluation is initiated from the "up" position (hands are shoulder-width apart, back is straight, and head is in neutral position). The individual is informed that they are not allowed to have their feet against a wall or other stationary item. Additionally, the individual is informed that the back must be straight at all times and they must push up to a straight arm position. The individual is instructed to continue performing push-ups in time with the cadence of the metronome, one beat up and one beat down. Inform the individual that if at any time during the evaluation they experience chest pain, light-headedness, ataxia, confusion, nausea, or clamminess, they should terminate the evaluation.

3. The evaluator places the five-inch prop on the ground beneath the individual's chin and the individual must lower the body to the floor until the chin touches this object.

4. The metronome should be set at a speed of 80, allowing for 40 push-ups per minute.

5. The individual has a two-minute time limit to complete a maximum of 80 push-ups.

6. The administrator shall stop the evaluation when the individual:

   a. Reaches 80 push-ups;

   b. Performs three consecutive incorrect push-ups; or

   c. Does not maintain continuous motion with the metronome cadence.

7. Record the highest number of successfully completed push-ups.

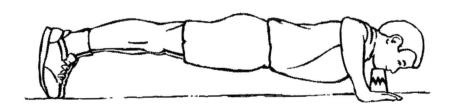

CURL-UP

Wellness-Fitness Initiative Curl-up Evaluation Protocol

Equipment

Gym mat
Metronome
Stopwatch

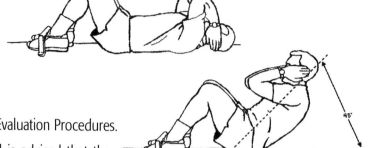

Protocol

1. Conduct Pre-Evaluation Procedures.

2. The individual is advised that the evaluation is a series of curl-ups performed in a three-minute time period. The individual is informed that the evaluation is initiated from the supine position with knees bent at a 90-degree angle, hands cupped over the ears or at the temples, and with hand and arm position maintained for the entire duration of the evaluation. The individual is advised that his or her feet will be secured by a bar or a second administrator, but the holding or bracing of the knees and or ankles is not allowed. The individual is instructed that the curl-up is initiated by flattening the lower back followed by actively contracting the abdominal muscles and then continuing the movement until the trunk reaches a 45-degree angle with respect to the floor. This is followed by curling down of the trunk with the lower back fully contacting the mat before the upper back and shoulders. A rocking or bouncing movement is not permitted and the buttocks must remain in contact with the mat at all times. The individual is instructed to continue performing curl-ups in time with the cadence of the metronome, one beat up and one beat down. Inform the individual that if at any time during the evaluation they experience back pain, chest pain, light-headedness, ataxia, confusion, nausea, or clamminess, they should terminate the evaluation.

3. The metronome is set at a speed of 60, allowing for 30 curl-ups per minute.

4. The individual has a three-minute time limit to successfully complete a maximum of 90 curl-ups.

5. The administrator shall observe the evaluation from the side to ensure that each curl-up is performed correctly and shall stop the evaluation when the individual:

   a. Reaches 90 curl-ups;

   b. Performs three consecutive incorrect curl-ups; or

   c. Does not maintain continuous motion with the metronome cadence.

6. Record the highest number of successfully completed curl-ups.

FLEXIBILITY EVALUATION

Wellness-Fitness Initiative Sit and Reach Protocol

Equipment

Novel Acuflex I or equivalent trunk flexibility tester

Protocol

1. Conduct Pre-Evaluation Procedures.

2. The individual is advised that the evaluation is a series of three measurements that will evaluate the flexibility of the lower back, hamstring muscles, and shoulders. The individual is informed that the flexion required during this evaluation must be smooth and slow, as the individual advances the slide on the box to the most distal position possible. Inform the individual that if at any time during the evaluation they experience back pain, chest pain, light-headedness, ataxia, confusion, nausea, or clamminess, they should terminate the evaluation.

3. The individual is instructed to sit on the floor ensuring the head, upper back, and lower back are in contact with the wall. The individual is instructed to place legs together, fully extended. The sit and reach box with the sliding measurement guide is placed with the box flat against the feet.

4. While maintaining head and upper/lower back contact with the wall, the individual is instructed to extend arms fully in front of the body with the right hand overlaying the left hand, with middle finger of each hand directly over each other. The rule is set to 0.0 inches at the tips of the middle fingers. The individ-ual is then instructed to exhale slowly while stretching slowly forward, bending at the waist and pushing the measuring device with the middle fingers. During the stretch, legs are to remain together and fully extended and hands are to remain overlaid. The stretch is held momentarily and the distance obtained. If the individual bounces, flexes the knees, or uses momentum to increase distance, the evaluation is not counted.

5. Instruct the individual to relax for 30 seconds. Once the individual has completed the 30-second recovery period begin the second evaluation. Repeat evaluation for the third time using the same procedure.

6. Record the furthest distance from the three trials (rounded to the nearest 1/4 inch) as the final score.

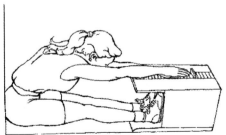

FITNESS EVALUATION EQUIPMENT LIST

- LifeFitness 9100HR Treadmill

  For Information and Local Distributor contact:

  LifeFitness
  10601 West Belmont Avenue
  Franklin Park IL 60131
  Phone: (847) 288-3300
  FAX: (847) 288-3791
  Web site: www.lifefitness.com

- Jackson Strength Evaluation System with V-Grip Handlebar (chinning triangle)*

  For Information and Local Distributor contact:

  Lafayette Instrument
  3700 Sagamore Parkway North
  P.O. Box 5729
  Lafayette, Indiana 47903
  Phone: (765) 423-1505 or
  (800) 428-7545
  FAX: (765) 423-4111
  Web site: www.licmef.com

- Jamar Hydraulic Hand Dynamometer*

  For Information and Local Distributor contact:

  Jamar Sammons Preston
  4 Sammons Court
  Bolingbrook, IL 60440
  Phone: (800) 323-5547

*Note: The Jackson Strength Evaluation System includes a Jamar Hydraulic Hand Dynamometer

- Novel Acuflex I Trunk Flexibility Tester

  For Information and Local Distributor contact:

  Novel Products Incorporated
  Post Office 408
  Rockton, Illinois 61072-0408
  Phone: (800) 323-5143
  FAX: 815-624-4866
  E-mail: novelprod@aol.com

- Polar Heart Rate Monitor

  For Information and Local Distributor contact:

  Polar Electro Inc.
  370 Crossways Park Drive
  Woodbury, New York 11797
  Phone: (800) 227-1314;
  Canada (888) 918-5043
  FAX: (516) 364-5454
  Web site: www.polarus.com

- StairMaster StepMill 7000 PT

  For Information and Local Distributor contact:

  StairMaster Sports/Medical Products, Inc.
  1886 Prairie Way
  Louisville, CO 80027
  Phone: (800) 782-4799
  Web site: www.stairmaster.com

FITNESS PROTOCOL WORKSHEET

Name:_____ Date: _____

Last Medical Exam Date: _____ Weight: _____ kg (*1 lb. = .45 kg*)

Age: _____

Resting Heart Rate: _____ *(If greater than 110 bpm, provide 5-minute rest; if after rest heart rate is greater than 110 bpm postpone evaluation)*

Resting Blood Pressure: _____ *(If greater than 160/100, provide 5-minute rest; if after rest blood pressure is greater than 160/100 postpone evaluation)*

Target Exercise Heart Rate _____ [.85(220–age)]

AEROBIC CAPACITY EVALUATION – GERKIN PROTOCOL

Uniformed personnel's heart rate is monitored continuously throughout the evaluation and during the cool-down period. Heart rate is obtained during the final 15 seconds of each stage and recorded. Once the individual's heart rate exceeds the target exercise heart rate, the individual continues the evaluation for an additional 15 seconds at the stage where the target exercise heart rate was exceeded. The evaluation is completed and the final evaluation stage is reported if the heart rate does not return to, or below, the target exercise heart rate or the individual reaches stage 11.4. The $\dot{V}O_2$max is determined by using the obtained final evaluation stage and the conversion chart. Record the heart rate after one minute of cool-down.

Stage 1: 4.5 mph, 0% grade Heart Rate: _____

Stage 2: 4.5 mph, 2% grade Heart Rate: _____

Stage 3: 5.0 mph, 2% grade Heart Rate: _____

Stage 4: 5.0 mph, 4% grade Heart Rate: _____

Stage 5: 5.5 mph, 4% grade Heart Rate: _____

Stage 6: 5.5 mph, 6% grade Heart Rate: _____

Stage 7: 6.0 mph, 6% grade Heart Rate: _____

Stage 8: 6.0 mph, 8% grade Heart Rate: _____

Stage 9: 6.5 mph, 8% grade Heart Rate: _____

Stage 10: 6.5 mph, 10% grade Heart Rate: _____

Stage 11: 7.0 mph, 10% grade Heart Rate: _____

Stage completed: _____

Converted $\dot{V}O_2$max: _____ ml/kg/min (see page 74 for Conversion Table)

Time evaluation terminated: _____, give reason(s).

Heart rate after one minute of cool-down period: _____

AEROBIC CAPACITY EVALUATION – FDNY PROTOCOL

Uniformed personnel's heart rate is monitored continuously throughout the evaluation. Heart rate is as obtained during the final 15 seconds of the evaluation and recorded.

Final Heart Rate: _____

The following equations are used to establish $\dot{V}O_2max$:

Male $\dot{V}O_2max = 113.34 - .15$ (weight) $- .32$ (final heart rate) $- .54$ (age)

Female $\dot{V}O_2max = 88.22 - .31$ (final heart rate) $- .32$ (age)

$\dot{V}O_2max$: _____ ml/kg/min

Time evaluation terminated: _____, give reason(s): _____

STRENGTH EVALUATION – GRIP

Dominant Hand: _____ Left / _____ Right

Trial 1, Left Hand: _____ kilograms   Trial 1, Right Hand: _____ kilograms

Trial 2, Left Hand: _____ kilograms   Trial 2, Right Hand: _____ kilograms

Trial 3, Left Hand: _____ kilograms   Trial 3, Right Hand: _____ kilograms

Highest Grip Strength Score: _____ kilograms

Evaluation terminated, give reason(s): _____

STRENGTH EVALUATION – LEG

Trial 1: _____ kilograms

Trail 2: _____ kilograms

Trial 3: _____ kilograms

Highest Leg Strength Score: _____ kilograms

Evaluation terminated, give reason(s): _____

STRENGTH EVALUATION – ARM

Trial 1: _____ kilograms

Trial 2: _____ kilograms

Trial 3: _____ kilograms

Highest Arm Strength Score: _____ kilograms

Evaluation terminated, give reason(s): _____

ENDURANCE EVALUATION – PUSH-UP

Number of successfully completed push-ups: _____

Evaluation terminated, give reason(s): _____

ENDURANCE EVALUATION – CURL-UP

Number of successfully completed curl-ups: _____

Evaluation terminated, give reason(s): _____

FLEXIBILITY EVALUATION – SIT AND REACH

Trial 1: _____ inches

Trial 2: _____ inches

Trial 3: _____ inches

Furthest distance: _____ inches

Evaluation terminated, give reason(s): _____

SELF-ASSESSMENT PROTOCOL

EXAMPLE OF CIRCUIT SELF-ASSESSMENT TEST

Note: The uniformed personnel should be properly warmed-up and medically cleared to participate in this evaluation. Once the test has begun, the individual should move from one station to the next with no more than 30 seconds between events. Movements with weights should be through the full range of motion, and include both the concentric and eccentric contractions.

PROTOCOL

1. Prior to performing the self evaluation, assemble the following equipment:

   Polar Heart Rate Monitor
   Dumbbells (pairs of 15 lbs., 20 lbs., 30 lbs., and 35 lbs.)
   Treadmill (capable of 5 mph and 15% grade)
   Lat Pulldown machine (set at 80 lbs)
   Flat Bench

2. Place equipment conveniently close to the treadmill since you will be returning to this piece of equipment.

3. Wet Polar Heart Receiver and put on chest. Tighten to a comfortable setting.

4. Turn on Polar watch and be sure it is receiving your heart rate.

5. Now you are ready to begin the evaluation. Remember that you will be recording both your time and your heart rate. Therefore you should move at as brisk a pace as you feel comfortable between events.

6. Get your self evaluation worksheet and mark the date. Keep this sheet with you as you proceed so you can record your heart rate immediately after each event.

7. Straddle the treadmill and start the belt. Be sure to set the exercise time for 20 minutes so it can run continually during your evaluation. Set the speed for 3.5 mph while you increase the incline to 15%. As soon as the belt reaches two mph, you can step on the treadmill. Once the incline reaches 15%, increase the speed to 5.0 mph. As soon as the speed hits 5.0 mph, begin timing your evaluation.

8. You will run on the treadmill @ 5.0 mph @ 15% grade for one minute. At the end of one minute, reduce the speed to 3.5 mph and step off the treadmill. Record your heart rate and move to the 15 lb. dumbbells.

9. Pick up the 15 lb. dumbbells and perform 24 biceps curls with both arms simultaneously. Do not swing your arms or upper body. Be sure to move through the full range of motion. After the 24th repetition, record your heart rate and move back to the treadmill.

10. Walk on the treadmill for 1 minute @ 3.5 mph @ 15% grade. At the completion of one minute, record your heart rate and move onto the dumbbell row.

11. Place your left knee and left arm on the flat bench and pick up the 30 lb. dumbbell with your right hand. Keeping your chest parallel to the ground, pull the dumbbell upward and into your lower chest. Perform 24 repetitions with your right arm and then repeat with your left arm. Record your heart rate and move onto the treadmill.

12. Walk on the treadmill for one minute @ 3.5 mph @ 15% grade. At the completion of one minute record your heart rate and move onto the dumbbell military press.

13. Pick up the 20 lb. dumbbells and, in a standing position, perform 24 repetitions (with each arm) of alternating military press. Record your heart rate and move onto the treadmill.

14. Walk on the treadmill for one minute @ 3.5 mph @ 15% grade. At the completion of one minute, record your heart rate and move onto the dumbbell carry.

15. Bend down using your legs and pickup both 35 lb. dumbbells (one in each hand). Carry the dumbbells to a mark six feet away and set them down on the ground. Turn, pick up the dumbbells and return to the starting line. Repeat this for 10 repetitions. Each time you set down the dumbbells is one repetition. Record your heart rate and return to the treadmill.

16. Walk on the treadmill for one minute @ 3.5 mph @ 15% grade. At the completion of one minute, record your heart rate and move onto the lat pulldown.

Name: _____

Target Exercise Heart Rate: _____

Date:					
Exercise	Heart Rate	Heart Rate	Heart Rate	Heart Rate	Heart Rate
Treadmill @ 15% @ 5 mph for 1 min.					
DB Curls @ 15 lbs, 24 reps (standing - both arms)					
Treadmill @ 15% @ 3.5 mph for 1 min.					
DB Rows @ 30 lbs, 24 reps (each arm)					
Treadmill @ 15% @ 3.5 mph for 1 min.					
DB Military Press @ 20 lbs, 24 reps (standing - alternating arms)					
Treadmill @ 15% @ 3.5 mph for 1 min.					
DB Carry @ 35 lbs, 10 reps (pick-up/carry six feet)					
Treadmill @ 15% @ 3.5 mph for 1 min.					
Lat Pulldown @ 80 lbs, 24 reps (close grip/palms toward face)					
1 minute of recovery (sitting quietly)					
2 minutes of recovery (sitting quietly)					
3 minutes of recovery (sitting quietly)					
4 minutes of recovery (sitting quietly)					
5 minutes of recovery (sitting quietly)					

17. Sit down with knees secured and grasp the straight lat pulldown bar with your hands close together and your palms supinated so they are facing you. Pull down in front of your body until the bar reaches your chin. Perform 24 repetitions, being sure to go all the way up. Record your total time and heart rate.

18. Sit in a quiet location and record your heart rate every minute for five minutes.

INTERPRETING YOUR RESULTS

1. Determine 85% of your estimated maximum heart rate, which will be the target exercise heart rate, using the following simple Karvonen Method equation:

   Target exercise heart rate = .85 (220 − age)
   Example: The target exercise heart rate of a 40-year-old individual is:
   Target exercise heart rate = .85 (220 − 40) = 153

2. Observe your heart rate throughout the test and see if it ever goes over your 85% value. If your heart rate is near maximal, it may indicate that you need to work on your cardiovascular conditioning. This indicates that you have very little reserve if some greater demand occurred on the fireground.

3. Observe each event and see if you completed the required number of repetitions. If you could not complete the required number of repetitions, you need to work on your muscular strength and/or endurance in these muscle groups.

4. Observe your total time and compare it to your last total time. If your total time for this test is less than your last test and your heart rate response is the same or less, your fitness level has improved.

5. Observe your five-minute recovery. A heart rate that recovers quickly is indicative of aerobic fitness. If your five-minute heart rate is less than your last test, your fitness level has improved.

REFERENCES

Brzycki, M. (1993) Strength testing: predicting a one-rep max from reps to fatigue. *JOPERD*, 64, 88-90.

National Strength and Conditioning Association. (2000). *Essentials of Strength Training and Conditioning*, Baechle, T. R. & Earle, R. W., eds. Champaign, Ill.: Human Kinetics.

FIRE FIGHTER INJURY
PREVENTION
GUIDELINES

FIRE FIGHTER INJURY PREVENTION

Every year, death and injury statistics show what fire fighters across North America already know – firefighting is one of the most hazardous occupations. The U.S. Fire Administration (USFA), National Institute of Occupational Safety and Health (NIOSH), the National Fire Protection Association (NFPA), and the International Association of Fire Fighters (IAFF) all concur that action must be taken to make the job safer. The statistic that every year one out of every three fire fighters will become injured has been heard so many times that it is almost accepted as the norm. The IAFF/IAFC Joint Labor Management Wellness-Fitness Initiative, NFPA 1710 Deployment Standard, and the NIOSH Fire fighter Fatality Reports are all efforts to change these statistics (Figures 5.1 and 5.2).

Figure 5.1

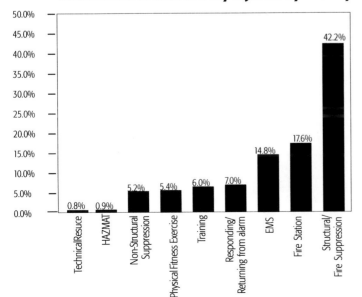

Distribution of Line of Duty Injuries by Activity

CHAPTER

5

Figure 5.2

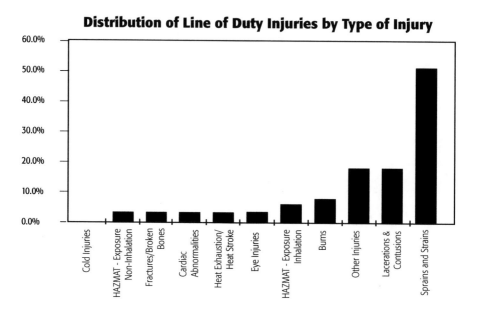

There is no magic bullet to prevent all fire fighter deaths and injuries. The answer lies in a change in the philosophy and culture of the fire service where safety and prevention become the models of professionalism. This chapter will look at a few ways that PFTs can help prevent fire fighter injuries.

ERGONOMICS

The science of making the work environment safer and more productive is called ergonomics. In order to understand the PFT's role in preventing injuries, you must first understand how ergonomics affects the fire service (Table 5.1).

The first step in reducing the number and severity of injuries is to perform an ergonomic hazard assessment. This assessment identifies and evaluates general workplace ergonomic risks. Many different specialists contribute to an assessment, including industrial hygienists, industrial safety officers, occupational therapists, kinesiologists, and exercise physiologists.

Once the ergonomic hazard assessment is complete, a specialist may be consulted to analyze the report and provide recommendations. These recommendations usually address injuries common to fire fighters, correctable causes of these injuries, and solutions to prevent future injuries.

A number of fire fighter activities are easily targeted for an analysis of ergonomic hazards and these are discussed next.

Table 5.1 General Workplace Ergonomic Risks

1. **Forceful exertions**
   - ➢ Lower back – lifting heavy objects away from the body
   - ➢ Arm/hand – pinch grip, forced or prolonged and repeated deviation at wrist

2. **Awkward positions**
   - ➢ Spinal rotation under power
   - ➢ Shoulder elevations under power
   - ➢ Prolonged seated work
   - ➢ Elbows elevated
   - ➢ Deviated wrists

3. **Localized contact stress**
   - ➢ Body part contacts unpadded sharp edge
   - ➢ Grasping small diameter tools
   - ➢ Using body part as striking tool

4. **Vibration**
   - ➢ Extended operation of power hand tools
   - ➢ Heavy equipment vibration

5. **Environmental conditions**
   - ➢ Heat – heat stress/hyperthermia
   - ➢ Cold – cold stress/hypothermia, reduced dexterity and tactility, frostbite
   - ➢ Particulate agents – smoke, dust, snow, sleet, etc.
   - ➢ Noise
   - ➢ Liquid and gaseous agents

6. **Repetitive/prolonged activity**
   - ➢ Tasks with short cycle times

Forceful Exertions

Fire fighters are frequently injured when lifting or carrying fire hoses, equipment, ladders, or victims. Some of these injuries occur outside the fire ground and may not involve emergency conditions. When lifting heavy objects, the fire fighter must make every effort to use the muscles of the lower body while maintaining a straight back and keeping the weight close to the body. Ideally, the fire fighter should lift heavy objects only from his or her safety zone. This zone is defined as the area close to the body from the waist to the shoulder. To reduce exposure to injuries from lifting heavy objects from low surfaces, heavy objects that are routinely lifted can be stored in accessible areas approximately three to four feet from the walking surface.

Improperly designed tools that must be carried to and from the scene can be difficult to transport or use. More attention must be placed on the design and correct ergonomic use of these items.

Awkward Positions

Fire fighters and EMTs must routinely assume awkward positions. For example, in fire suppression keeping low to the ground to avoid rising heat and the hot temperatures in a room or removing victims from cramped spaces cluttered with debris. On vehicle accidents, fire fighters and EMTs must often use extrication equipment and remove victims while bent over on uneven surfaces.

Emergency medical workers provide patient care at the site of the emergency, often involving improper and uneven work surfaces or difficult environmental conditions. Injuries may occur because of the weight shift as the rescuer is required to support a patient's body weight while working on irregular surfaces. Improving the muscular strength of the back, abdominals, and legs may enable personnel to better compensate for weight shifts and ultimately reduce the risk of injury.

A significant number of injuries occur during vehicular use. Step heights must be considered as well as the riding position of the fire fighter when going to or returning from emergency scenes. The risk of injuries from stepping off the fire apparatus can be reduced by providing handrails on the apparatus so that fire fighters can support themselves as they mount and dismount the apparatus. Training fire fighters in proper dismounting techniques that reduce the forces placed on the body can also reduce the risk of injury.

Environmental Conditions

Fire fighter protective clothing and equipment can reduce mobility, hand dexterity, and tactility while adding to the workload. This can lead to heat stress, which can progress to heat exhaustion and life-threatening heat stroke if not properly managed.

COMMON INJURIES

The three most common musculoskeletal injuries fire fighters experience are: back, shoulder, and knee injuries. To design a prevention program, you must understand the common ergonomic and anatomical causes (Table 5.2).

Table 5.2 Ergonomic and Anatomical Causes of Injury

	Causes	Prevention
Lower Back Injuries		
Ergonomic	1. Forceful Exertions – lifting heavy objects away from the body and in excess of physical capacity 2. Operating in awkward postures – spinal rotation while under load, bending over at the waist to operate at ground level, picking up equipment from high or low locations	1. Get help lifting heavy objects when possible. 2. Use proper lifting technique by keeping heavy objects as close to the center of gravity of the lifter's body 3. Identify awkward positions and compensate by using more people to share load 4. Avoid bending at the waist and instead bend the knees, crouch down, or sit down
Anatomic	1. Weak leg, back, and abdominal muscles 2. Poor hamstring flexibility 3. Obesity	1. Perform functionally consistent strength training to improve muscular strength and endurance 2. Stretch regularly with an emphasis on slow, static hamstring stretches 3. Engage in a comprehensive weight management program
Shoulder Injuries		
Ergonomic	1. Forceful exertions – lifting heavy objects overhead without support, lifting heavy objects without warm-up 2. Awkward postures – shoulder elevations while under load, swinging hand tools in limited visibility, operating overhead in vulnerable positions 3. Environmental conditions – personal protective equipment (PPE) presents additional stress on shoulder joint from weight of equipment & SCBA 4. Repetitive/prolonged activity – operating with arms above head for prolonged periods of time	1. Get help when lifting heavy objects; warm-up shoulders prior to heavy exertion 2. Learn limitations and avoid over-swinging tools; when operating overhead, attempt to adjust position frequently and when possible avoid fatigue 3. Look for lighter and more flexible PPE 4. Frequently rotate crewmembers to avoid undue fatigue
Anatomic	1. Weak rotator cuff muscles 2. Anterior-to-posterior strength imbalance 3. Shoulder girdle laxity 4. Lack of shoulder girdle flexibility	1. Perform consistent strength training 2. Strengthen posterior muscles of shoulder girdle 3. Strengthen muscles surrounding the shoulder girdle, especially the stabilizers 4. Consistently stretch shoulder girdle muscles
Knee Injuries		
Ergonomic	1. Forceful exertions – attempting to lift objects heavier than capacity 2. Awkward postures – operating on uneven surfaces while under load 3. Localized contact stress – foot planted	1. Strengthen leg muscles using primarily closed-chain exercises 2. Perform proprioceptive functional exercises 3. Identify high-risk situations and get help when needed
Anatomic	1. Weak knee stabilizers	1. Strengthen leg muscles using primarily closed-chain exercises 2. Perform proprioceptive functional exercises 3. Strengthen muscles of lower extremity

FIRE FIGHTER HEAT STRESS AND HYDRATION

Fire fighters working in heated environments generate body heat rapidly in the process of supplying energy to active muscles. Fire Fighters also absorb heat energy from exposure to active flames, hot gases, and heated surfaces. Protective gear insulates the fire fighter, and if the work environment is hotter than skin temperature, heat can only be dissipated through the evaporation of sweat. Because humans tend to gain heat faster than can be lost, heat energy accumulates, causing the body temperature to rise. Blood is redirected to the skin and sweat is produced to facilitate cooling. Both of these actions reduce the body's ability to perform at top efficiency and decrease work capacity. Progressive heat gain and body fluid loss can produce dangerous conditions of hyperthermia and dehydration and increases the risk of heat illness and injury (Table 5.3). Properly hydrated, well-conditioned fire fighters are better able to contend with heat stress than their unconditioned counterparts. The notion that limiting fluid intake during workouts will help "toughen-up" athletes is a dangerous, archaic misconception.

Table 5.3 Symptoms of Dehydration

Early Signs	Severe Signs
Fatigue	Difficulty swallowing
Headache	Stumbling
Flushed skin	Clumsiness
Burning in stomach	Sunken eyes and dim vision
Light-headedness	Painful urination
Dark urine	Dark urine with a strong odor
Dry mouth	Numb skin
Dry cough	Muscle spasms
Heat intolerance	Delirium
Loss of appetite	

Chronic, mild dehydration and poor fluid intake may influence the following health and performance factors (Kleiner, 1999):

*Diminished physical performance

*Diminished mental performance

*Diminished salivary gland function

*Increased risk of kidney stones in susceptible individuals

*Increased risk of urinary tract cancers

*Increased risk of colon cancer

*Increased risk of breast cancer

*Increased risk of childhood obesity

*Increased risk of mitral valve prolapse in susceptible individuals

ACCLIMATIZATION

Ideally, athletes train in environments similar to those in which they will perform. Conversely, individuals who exercise exclusively in cool, air-conditioned environments are physically and psychologically disadvantaged when forced to perform in hot environments.

Repeated exposure to heat results in adaptive physiological changes that improve performance in hot environments. Individuals who have become acclimatized to hot environments sweat more, sweat sooner, and better preserve electrolytes, resulting in greater heat dissipation and lower skin and core temperatures.

While consistent cardiovascular training provides some improvement in heat tolerance, and exposures to hot environments (without exercising) will also result in some degree of acclimatization, systematic, graduated exercise programs in hot environments achieve the most substantial improvements relatively quickly. Cardiovascular changes occur within three to five days. However, sweating mechanisms require up to 10 days to reach peak acclimatization. During the acclimatization period, daily heat exposure of two to four hours is recommended. The first two or three exercise sessions should be reduced in intensity to 60 to 70% of maximum capacity. After these initial sessions, exercise intensity should be increased gradually. It is imperative that pre-hydration, fluid intake during exercise, and rehydration be emphasized. This period can serve as useful education, helping individuals learn beverage preferences and rehydration capabilities. Note that positive benefits of acclimatization are transient, and are lost two to three weeks after heat exposure ceases.

Individuals may lose body fluids at somewhat higher or lower rates depending upon body size and individual sweat capacity. On average, working fire fighters should anticipate losing between 1.5 to 2.0 liters of sweat in a 30 to 45 minute operation (Levine et al., 1990). Studies have indicated that in a 30- to 45-minute workout performed at 60% of maximal intensity in hot, humid temperatures, approximately 2% of body weight can be lost (Sawka & Pandolf, 1990; Craig & Cummings, 1966). For a 200-pound fire fighter, a 2% sweat-induced loss of body weight would require a post-exercise fluid intake of about 2.8 liters (12 cups) or more. To minimize heat illness and injury potential, fire fighters must cool themselves off and replenish their fluid loss immediately after concluding work assignments (Table 5.4).

Dehydration impairs perception of effort, cardiovascular function, ability to dissipate heat, and physical work capacity. Gradual fluid loss may proceed undetected, because the sensation of thirst may not be triggered until water deficits reach 1 to 2% of body weight. A seemingly minor drop in body hydration can have a dramatic impact on performance. A loss of 2% of weight through dehydration can diminish performance by 10 to 15%. Fire fighters must avoid being placed in the dangerous position of entering fire situations when poorly hydrated.

Once a fire fighter has been relieved from assignment at an emergency operation, further body fluid loss must be limited and the fire fighter must begin to re-hydrate. To reduce the rate of sweating, allow the body to cool off by moving to a shaded area and remove equipment, bunker gear, helmet, hood, and gloves. Cool water spray and exposure to forced air or wind accelerate the process of cooling.

It is highly recommended that hydration level be monitored frequently. Two methods for daily evaluation of personal hydration are described below. The thirst mechanism is inadequate to indicate hydration, because individuals do not develop the sensation of thirst until they are significantly dehydrated. By the time the brain gets the signal of thirst, 1% of body weight has been lost.

Table 5.4 Fluid Intake Guidelines

Did you know that one gulp is about one ounce?			
Daily	Before Exercise	During Exercise	After Exercise
❑ At least eight 8-oz. cups ❑ Minimum 1 quart (32 ounces) for each 1,000 calories intake ❑ By the time the brain gets the thirst signal, 1% of body weight has been lost. ❑ A 2% weight loss due to dehydration will cut performance by 10–15%. ❑ Fluids should be cool (40–50° F), & ingested regularly throughout the day. ❑ Avoid caffeine, alcohol and high sugar fluids.	**Light Exercise**		
	2 hours before exercise consume at least 16 oz. 15–30 minutes before exercise, consume an additional 8 oz. of fluid	6–11 oz. every 15–20 minutes or 21–43 oz. per hour during exercise	Depending on length of exercise, intensity, body weight, environmental temperature, etc., as much as 64–96 oz. (8–12 cups) of fluid per hour of exercise should be ingested for optimal recovery.
	Moderate Exercise		
	For moderate exercise that lasts an hour or less, water is sufficient for replacing lost fluids. If flavored drinks are desired, then use lightly flavored, non-caffeinated, non-carbonated beverages.		
	Intense Exercise		
	For intense exercise that lasts less than 1 hour or any exercise lasting more than 90 minutes, 6–8% carbohydrate-electrolyte sport drinks or diluted juices are best. Some people have gastrointestinal problems after ingesting drinks with high concentrations of fructose during exercise. Avoid caffeinated drinks during and after workouts. Choose a beverage with a small amount (.5–1 gram per liter) of sodium. Electrolyte replacement is important for re-hydration since loss of up to 1 gram of sodium per hour of exercise can occur.		

MORNING HYDRATION MAINTENANCE
A. Urinate; B. Monitor Body Weight; C. Re-hydrate

One way to monitor daily state of hydration is body weight. For three to four mornings in a row, the fire fighter should monitor body weight after urinating. This will establish the baseline "normal" body weight. Weight should be checked first thing each morning using the same scale and wearing approximately the same amount of clothing. If weight has dropped by 2 to 4 pounds compared to the last few weigh-ins, the weight lost is likely an indication of water loss (dehydration). For each pound of water weight lost, consume at least 16 to 20 ounces (or at least one-and-a-half times as much fluid as has been lost) of water, or non-caffeinated, alcohol-free beverage *in addition to daily fluid intake.*

Monitor Urine Color

Evaluation of hydration level by weight is less reliable throughout the day, because body weight can fluctuate independent of hydration level, meals, and other variables. The best bet is to start the day well hydrated and observe urine color. Urine should be light (straw) colored or clear. Dark (amber) urine with an odor is a sign of dehydration. Continue to take in fluids via appropriate beverages, fruits, and vegetables throughout the day and minimize or eliminate intake of alcohol and caffeine.

COUNTERMEASURE TO ENSURE PROPER HYDRATION

An effective way to delay the onset of dehydration is to increase total body water. There is a 10 to 12% increase in blood plasma volume associated with regular physical exercise. Consistent aerobic training results in increased efficiency, effectiveness, and absolute capacity of the body's cooling mechanisms. The better-conditioned fire fighters will carry more water and lose fewer electrolytes via sweat, thus enabling them to re-hydrate quickly and completely. Muscle mass is relatively high in water content (about 75%), compared to fat (generally less than 25%). So, the leaner the individual, the greater his or her body water stores.

To achieve an optimal rate of re-hydration, fire fighters should drink fluids that are cold (40° to 50°F; 4.4° to 10°C), dilute, and carbohydrate-based with a small measure of sodium. Sodium, an electrolyte, can be lost through sweat at a rate of 1 gram or more per hour of heavy exercise. Sodium makes the drink more palatable and aids in fluid retention. The sodium content of juices is only about 20 mg per liter. Sports drinks have about 100 to 700 mg of sodium per liter. For optimal rehydration, 0.5 to 1 gram of sodium per liter of fluid is recommended. During exercise, carbohydrates are absorbed into the bloodstream at the rate of about 1 gram per minute (60 g/hr). Sports drinks contain between 50 and 80 grams of carbohydrate per liter.

It takes at least 64 to 96 ounces of fluid, or 8 to12 cups, to replace fluid loss of 1.5 to 2.0 liters. This is equivalent to consuming at least one-and-a-half times as much fluid as has been lost. Rapid re-hydration can be accomplished by mixing juice with an equal quantity of chilled tap water or by drinking a commercial sports drink. Ideally, drink enough to fill your stomach to about 75% of capacity (about 0.6 liters or 2.5 cups) and continue to top fluids off at that level by consuming an additional 6 to 8 ounces (3/4 to 1 cup) of fluid every 10 to 15 minutes. The body can only absorb approximately 2.4 liters per hour. Since individual rates of fluid absorption vary widely, use caution and monitor gastric comfort. Most people tend to consume smaller volumes at shorter intervals to avoid exercising or working with a full stomach.

It is counterproductive to consume beverages that are either hot or have high concentrations of sugars, protein, or fat. Such drinks stay in the stomach longer because they require more digestion time. Increased digestion time delays the passage of water into the small intestine, and its subsequent absorption into the blood stream.

For daily hydration and performance, fire fighters should choose foods from the carbohydrate family (fruits, vegetables, breads, cereals, rice, grains, and pasta). Carbohydrates serve as the primary fuel source for the performance of most fire fighting tasks and, in the case of fruits and vegetables, contain comparatively large quantities of water.

REFERENCES

Craig, E.N. & Cummings, E.G. (1966) Dehydration and muscular work. *J Appl Physiol,* 21, 670–4.

Kleiner, S.M. (1999). Water: An essential but overlooked nutrient. *J AM Diet Assoc,* 200–206.

Levine, L. et al. (1990). Physiologic strain associated with wearing toxic-environment protective systems during exercise in the heat. In: Das B., ed. *Advances in industrial ergonomics and safety II.* London: Taylor & Francis, 897–904.

Sawka, M.N. & Pandolf, K.B. (1990). Effects of body water loss on physiological function and exercise performance. In: Gisolfi, C.V. & Lamb, D.R., eds. *Perspectives in exercise science and sports medicine.* Vol. 3. Carmel, IN: Benchmark Press, 1–38.

IAFF/IAFC CANDIDATE
PHYSICAL ABILITY TEST

Across the United States and Canada, fire departments have been tasked by the legal challenges of hiring qualified fire fighters. In a proactive move, the IAFF and the IAFC collaborated to develop a comprehensive candidate physical ability test (CPAT) program. The test was created by a Task Force consisting of members from the IAFF and IAFC, the fire chiefs and their respective local union presidents from ten large metropolitan area fire departments, along with other technical experts. The IAFF/IAFC CPAT program ensures that new fire fighter candidates are physically capable of performing the challenging job of a fire fighter and making it possible to broaden the diversity of the fire service. The Task Force also worked closely with the U.S. Department of Justice throughout the development of a valid and functional candidate physical ability test.

The *CPAT Manual* provides instruction in administering the CPAT: developing recruiting and mentoring programs, preparing candidates to be successful, and setting up and administering the test. The entire validation process is discussed in detail, along with the legal issues that departments might face when implementing testing. The IAFF facilitated this effort and utilized its resources to provide fair and valid testing standards across the fire service. The IAFC's commitment and participation demonstrated a shared vision of excellence for the fire service.

The goal of the CPAT project remains the same as in the Fire Service Joint-Labor Management Wellness-Fitness Initiative – to improve the quality of life of all fire fighters. When diverse groups of physically qualified candidates become fire fighters, and then participate in comprehensive wellness/fitness programs, a win-win situation is created. Communities receive better service, fire departments improve performance, and the fire fighters enjoy long, healthy careers and retirements.

CHAPTER 6

The Task Force directed its technical committee to develop and validate a candidate physical ability test for the ten jurisdictions. The technical committee was instructed to develop a test that would measure a candidate's physical ability to perform the critical tasks of a fire fighter. The technical committee undertook the following steps in meeting the Task Force's directive:

1. Reviewed current job analysis, job descriptions, and existing physical ability tests in the represented jurisdictions to establish a list of essential tasks

2. Developed a survey to measure the criticality and physicality of essential tasks common to fire departments

3. Developed an equipment survey

4. Identified the total number of surveys to be distributed to each department as well as the number to be distributed to target minority groups within each department

5. Administered the surveys

6. Weighed and measured all standard firefighting equipment

7. Compiled and analyzed the survey responses

8. Reviewed data among departments as well as among all groups to determine whether any groups or departments were not the same

9. Reviewed equipment surveys to identify tools and equipment that were common between all departments

10. Analyzed data from surveys for criticality and physicality

11. Identified tasks as testable or non-testable

12. Developed pilot CPAT

13. Designed and built prototype props to simulate tasks chosen for the CPAT

14. Evaluated several orders of tasks within the CPAT and sequenced optimal order to avoid undue demands on applicants

15. Evaluated and redesigned props

16. Developed the final version of the CPAT

17. Developed an incumbent survey to measure the need for special skills, the quality of the props and simulations, and the content of the tasks chosen

18. Randomly selected incumbents to take the CPAT

19. Collected surveys completed by incumbents, compiled and analyzed data

20. Tested and surveyed 33 training experts from all ten consortium jurisdictions to measure the need for special skills, the quality of the props and simulations, and the content of the tasks chosen

21. Filmed fire fighters acting out the CPAT at various times

22. Developed pass/fail times by having training officers view videos of fire fighter performing at different times; officers evaluated times as acceptable, marginally acceptable, marginally unacceptable, or unacceptable

23. Collected, compiled, and analyzed data from training officers on video time ratings

24. Statistically developed fail times based on training officers' ratings

25. Presented data to Task Force for approval

26. Developed ways to proactively prevent unnecessary adverse impacts

27. Developed pre-test preparation time

28. Developed recruitment procedures

29. Developed orientation procedures

30. Developed test administration procedures

31. Developed validation document

32. Conducted an inter-rater reliability study to determine that trained Lead and Event Proctors could reproduce the results

33. Developed legal review document

The Fire Service Joint Labor Management Wellness Fitness Initiative's *CPAT Manual* has six major components:

1. Recruiting and Mentoring Physically Qualified Candidates

2. CPAT Preparatory Guide

3. CPAT Administration and Orientation

4. The Candidate Physical Ability Test

5. The CPAT Validation Process

6. Legal Issues

It should be noted that for a department to use the CPAT, all aspects of the *CPAT Manual* must be implemented. In addition, a transportability study must be administered prior to the implementation of the CPAT. Before administering the CPAT, it is imperative that the *CPAT Manual* be read in its entirety.

RECRUITING AND MENTORING

In today's society, communities are increasingly diverse and fire fighters are continually challenged to operate in multicultural environments. The fire department should reflect the community it serves. The objective of the CPAT is to test for those physically qualified to perform the job of a fire fighter. The CPAT cannot be separated from the department's broader goal of having a properly trained and physically capable workforce whose members reflect the diversity of the community. Diversity should be achieved by actively recruiting qualified men and women candidates from all ethnic backgrounds for careers in the fire service.

PFTs have a valuable role in recruiting and mentoring. Besides being role models, PFTs also have exposure to many diverse physically fit candidates. Whenever possible, PFTs should be involved with recruiting and mentoring efforts.

CANDIDATE PHYSICAL ABILITY TEST PREPARATION PROGRAM AND GUIDE

The U.S. Equal Employment Opportunity Commission and the Canadian Human Rights Commission recommends that employers provide all candidates with pretest materials to ensure that all candidates have equal opportunity to compete for the job of fire fighter. No one is more capable and qualified at leading preparatory programs than a PFT. Knowledge of physical fitness, combined with actual job experience, makes PFTs experts in how to prepare for the physical demands of fire fighting.

The preparation guide found in the *CPAT Manual* provides all candidates, regardless of their background or experience in exercise principles and techniques, the same opportunity to succeed. Distributing this preparation guide helps fire departments avoid failing candidates who are physically capable but unprepared for testing. The CPAT candidate preparation guide contains information on:

➤ The physical demands of the CPAT

➤ The necessity of proper hydration

➤ Basic training principles

➤ Warm-up techniques

➤ Flexibility techniques

➤ Muscular strength and endurance techniques

➤ Cardiovascular endurance techniques

➤ Training techniques for those without a gym or specialized equipment

All candidates should receive the preparation guide at least eight weeks prior to the CPAT date. The guide can be distributed at the time of application or at the orientation prior to the CPAT. In addition, departments may distribute the preparation guide during recruitment activities. Recent studies have shown that preparatory programs that last at least 12 weeks are more beneficial than programs that only last eight weeks. Therefore, PFTs should provide orientation and preparatory programs at least 12 weeks prior to the administration of the CPAT. More importantly, a preparatory program should continue beyond the CPAT to adequately prepare candidates for the Training Academy.

Fire departments should make reasonable efforts to provide free CPAT preparation opportunities. The CPAT preparation guide is a generic program developed for all potential candidates, but may require modification to improve its effectiveness for specific individuals. Preparatory programs can be developed and administered by the individual departments or cooperatively with other organizations, such as a local community college or YMCA. Many fire departments have used local community colleges to offer fire science, wellness, and exercise classes to help prepare future candidates for the job of fire fighter. Such resources may provide candidates who require additional time, or who need personalized instruction, better opportunities for success.

Successful preparatory programs should include:

- Educational materials and lessons on how and why to maintain fitness levels

- Specific workout programs to prepare for fire fighter job requirements

- Specific task oriented programs to prepare for the job of fire fighter (including, but not limited to, the CPAT events)

CPAT ADMINISTRATION AND ORIENTATION

Consistent test administration is essential to implementing a fair test to all candidates. Consistent test administration is achieved by using well-defined administration steps. The steps must follow the candidate from the time a test date is assigned to the completion of the CPAT. Each action by the department personnel administering a test should be clearly documented and followed without any deviation. Strict policies and procedures ensure that test administration is consistent from one candidate to another and avoids any biases. The CPAT administration guide to support the CPAT is found in Appendix 4-1 of the *CPAT Manual*, and includes information concerning how the test is administered:

- Logistical and environmental factors

- Venue and test props

- Scheduling, staging, and support

- Pre-test orientation

- Retesting

PRE-TEST ORIENTATION

It is essential to provide all candidates with an orientation on each element of the CPAT. This orientation introduces candidates to the test events and provides information on preparing physically for the job of fire fighter. This orientation should be provided by PFTs.

This orientation provides an opportunity for each candidate to view the test events, talk with instructors, and physically examine test equipment, tools, and props. Orientations are designed to give each candidate identical information regarding the test to maximize potential for testing success. The orientation guide to support this test is in Appendix 4-2 of the *CPAT Manual*.

During the pre-test orientation, PFTs explain the equipment used at that event, the purpose of that event, the event itself, and the failures associated with that event. In addition, PFTs explain the muscles and energy systems used and training tips for preparing for that event. Next, PFTs demonstrate the event along with the most common technique variations. Comments implying there is only one "correct" way to accomplish an event are usually inaccurate and suggest there is a learned skill for successful event completion. These types of comments should be avoided. To ensure consistency, PFTs should read this process from the materials in the *CPAT Manual*.

Once the event has been described and demonstrated, the candidates should be allowed to practice the event. During this practice time, PFTs should assist candidates to improve the effectiveness, efficiency, and safety of their techniques.

THE CPAT

The CPAT is a sequence of eight events that requires the candidate to progress along a predetermined path from event to event in a continuous manner. This is a pass/fail test based on a validated maximum total time of 10 minutes and 20 seconds.

In these events, the candidate wears a 50-pound vest to simulate the weight of self-contained breathing apparatus (SCBA) and fire fighter protective clothing. An additional 25 pounds, using two 12.5-pound weights that simulate a high-rise pack (hose bundle), is added for the stair climb event.

Throughout all events, the candidate must wear long pants, a hard hat with chinstrap, work gloves, and footwear with no open heel or toe. Watches and loose or restrictive jewelry are not permitted.

All props were chosen to provide the highest level of consistency, safety, and validity in measuring the candidate's physical abilities. Schematic drawings and specifications for each prop are included in Appendix 5 of the *CPAT Manual*. All props for the CPAT must be purchased through the vendors specified by the *CPAT Manual*. Modification of props or substitution of tools/equipment may alter the content of the test and therefore are not permitted. The entire test is designed to be portable and allow for either indoor or outdoor setup. The floor of the venue must be consistent for all events and for all candidates.

The events are placed in a sequence that best simulates their use in a fire scene while allowing for an 85-foot walk between events. To ensure the highest level of safety and prevent candidates from becoming exhausted, no running is allowed between events. This walk allows the candidate approximately 20 seconds to recover before each event.

To ensure scoring accuracy by eliminating timer failure, two stopwatches are used to time the CPAT. One stopwatch is designated as the official test time stopwatch; the second is the backup stopwatch. If mechanical failure occurs, the time on the backup stopwatch is used. The stopwatches are set to the past/fail time and countdown from 10 minutes and 20 seconds. If time elapses prior to the completion of the test, the test is concluded and the candidate fails the test.

The CPAT includes eight sequential events as follows:

1. Stair climbing
2. Hose drag
3. Equipment carry
4. Ladder raise and extension
5. Forcible entry
6. Search
7. Rescue
8. Ceiling breach and pull

Full descriptions of each event, including the required equipment, the purpose of the evaluation, the event itself, and performance deviations resulting in failure are found in the *CPAT Manual*.

CPAT VALIDATION PROCESS

The CPAT had to be validated before the Task Force could accept it as a legally defensible and legitimate tool for assessing fire fighter candidates. Any performance tests must meet validity criteria established by the Equal Employment Opportunity Commission (EEOC), United States Department of Justice (DOJ), United States Department of Labor (DOL), and the Canadian Human Rights Commission.

Briefly, there are three types of test validity:

1. *Content validity* determines that the elements of the test are similar to elements of the job.

2. *Criterion validity* uses advanced statistical techniques to show that the fitness tests predict job performance.

3. *Construct validity* describes the extent to which the test measures the underlying theoretical concepts and abilities related to the job.

Another validity concept of interest to the Task Force was the theory of validity transport. If a test is validated in one jurisdiction, based on a thorough job analysis and supported by a fairness study, it can be transported to another jurisdiction with the same job analysis. If the test is added to or changed between jurisdictions, however, the test is vulnerable to legal attack.

A valid candidate physical ability test yields results that meaningfully reflect a candidate's ability to perform the essential job duties of a fire fighter. It will also differentiate among candidates in their ability to perform the physically demanding tasks of a fire fighter.

LEGAL ISSUES

The *CPAT Manual* provides legal information regarding the CPAT in several key areas:

- ➢ Title VII Uniformed Hiring Guideline Requirements
- ➢ Transportability
- ➢ Adverse Impact
- ➢ Types of Validation
- ➢ Selection Procedures
- ➢ Cutoff Time Development
- ➢ Cutoff Time vs. Rank Order
- ➢ Documentation Requirements
- ➢ Fairness
- ➢ ADA Implications

Although much of this information is not part of the PFT's responsibility, the CPAT Administrator must be well versed on these issues.

CPAT — CANDIDATE PREPARATION GUIDE

The job of a fire fighter is one of the most physically demanding jobs in North America. It requires high levels of cardiopulmonary endurance, muscular strength, and muscular endurance. The Candidate Physical Ability Test consists of eight critical physical tasks that simulate actual job duties on the fireground. This test is physically demanding and requires that you be physically fit to be successful. This guide was developed to assist you with physically preparing yourself for the test.

What is physical fitness in the Fire Service?

Physical fitness is the ability to perform physical activities, such as job tasks, with enough reserve for emergency situations and to enjoy normal activities when off duty.

What are the major areas of fitness?

The major areas of physical fitness include:

- • flexibility
- • cardiopulmonary endurance
- • muscular strength
- • muscular endurance

Body composition is also considered an area of physical fitness. It should be noted that excess body fat increases the workload placed upon the body and decreases the body's ability to dissipate heat.

A proper physical fitness program should be specific to the job of a fire fighter. It should include all of the major areas of physical fitness mentioned above and be a total-body program. Although this is best accomplished at a gym with an array of equipment, this guide also includes exercises that require little or no equipment.

HYDRATION

Proper hydration is critical. All candidates should drink water before, during, and after exercise. Additionally, they should drink at least one liter of water one hour before the CPAT.

WARM-UP & FLEXIBILITY

A warm-up serves several functions, including:

- increased blood flow to working muscles and joints
- decreased likelihood of injury
- decrease in pre-event tension
- possible improved performance
- improved flexibility

A proper warm-up should begin with a few of minutes of the same type of activity you are about to do, but at a very light exertion level. For example, if you are preparing to go running, you should run in place or for a short distance at a very easy pace.

The next step is to stretch to improve flexibility and further your warm-up. There are two phases of stretching. The first phase is the easy stretch. In this phase, you should hold the stretch for 10 seconds in a range of motion that produces only mild tension. This prepares you for the second phase, the developmental stretch. In this phase, you should move slightly farther to the point where you feel a little more tension. This should be held for another 10 seconds.

FLEXIBILITY

When stretching, follow these basic rules:

- Stretch slowly
- No bouncing
- No pain
- Stretching is not competitive
- Breathe slowly to help you relax
- Stretching should feel good

STRETCHING EXERCISES

1. Knee to Chest

Glutes, Low Back, Hamstrings, Quadriceps

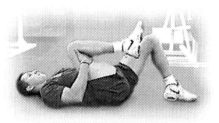

- Lay flat on your back with knees bent.

- Grab under the right thigh and pull knee toward chest until you feel mild tension.

- Hold for 10 seconds, then pull slightly farther until you feel slightly more tension.

- Hold this position for 10 seconds.

- Repeat with other leg.

- Repeat sequence 2 or 3 times.

2. Knee to Chest - Leg Straight

Glutes, Low Back, Hamstrings, Quadriceps

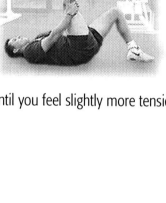

- Lay flat on your back with knees bent.

- Grab under the right thigh and straighten right leg. Do not lock knee.

- Hold for 10 seconds, then pull slightly farther until you feel slightly more tension.

- Hold this position for 10 seconds.

- Repeat with other leg.

- Repeat sequence 2 or 3 times.

3. Knee to Chest - Diagonal

Glutes, Low Back, Hamstrings, Quadriceps, Piriformis

- Lay flat on your back with knees bent.

- Grab under the right thigh and pull right knee toward left side of chest until you feel mild tension.

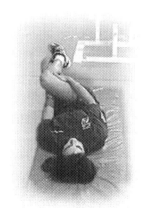

- Hold for 10 seconds, then pull slightly farther until you feel slightly more tension.

- Hold this position for 10 seconds.

- Repeat with other leg.

- Repeat sequence 2 or 3 times.

4. Leg Cross

Piriformis, Glutes, Low Back

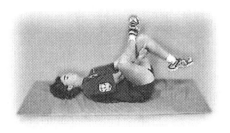

- Lay flat on your back with knees bent.
- Place your right outer ankle on the top of your left thigh.
- Grab under left thigh and pull left knee toward chest until you feel mild tension.
- Hold for 10 seconds, then pull slightly farther until you feel slightly more tension.
- Hold this position for 10 seconds.
- Repeat with other leg.
- Repeat sequence 2 or 3 times.

5. Side Quadricep Stretch

Quadriceps, Hip Flexors, Abdominals

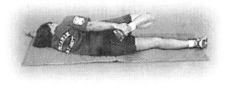

- Lay on your left side.
- Grab the right shin, just above your right ankle.
- Slowly pull right foot toward right buttock while pushing right hip forward.
- Hold for 10 seconds, then pull slightly farther until you feel slightly more tension.

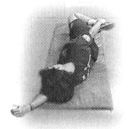

- Hold this position for 10 seconds.
- Repeat with other leg.
- Repeat sequence 2 or 3 times.

6. Butterfly Stretch

Groin, Low Back

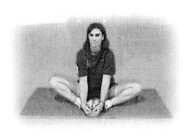

- Sit upright with the bottoms of your feet touching each other.
- Bend forward at the waist to a position where you feel mild tension.
- Elbows can be used to push down on thighs if you want more stretch.
- Hold for 10 seconds, then pull slightly farther until you feel slightly more tension.
- Hold this position for 10 seconds.
- Repeat sequence 2 or 3 times.

7. Straddle Stretch

Groin, Hamstrings, Low Back

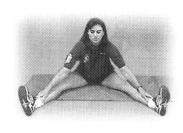

- Sit upright with legs straight.

- Spread legs as far as you comfortably can.

- Keeping legs straight, but not locking knees, bend forward at the waist.

- Hold for 10 seconds then push down slightly farther until you feel slightly more tension.

- Hold this position for 10 seconds.

- Return to starting position.

- Repeat sequence, but this time take chest toward left knee.

- Return to the starting position and repeat sequence toward right knee.

- Repeat entire sequence 2 or 3 times.

8. Cross Over Stretch

Glutes, Iliotibial Band

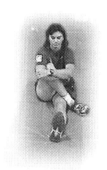

- Sit with legs straight in front of you.

- Bend right leg and cross it over so you can grab around the outside of right thigh.

- Slowly pull bent right leg toward chest until you feel mild tension.

- Hold for 10 seconds then push slightly farther until you feel slightly more tension.

- Hold this position for 10 seconds.

- Return to starting position and switch legs.

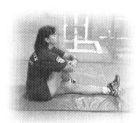

- Repeat sequence on opposite leg.

- Repeat sequence 2 or 3 times.

9. Calf Stretch

Calves

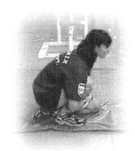

- Squat down on ground with right foot slightly in front of left.

- Grasp right shin and rock forward until you feel mild tension.

- Hold for 10 seconds, then push slightly farther until you feel slightly more tension.

- Hold this position for 10 seconds.

- Repeat sequence on opposite leg.

- Repeat sequence 2 or 3 times.

10. Upper Back Stretch

Upper Back, Posterior Deltoids

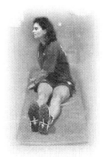

- Sit with legs straight in front.

- Twist your upper back, crossing the left arm across chest and place right hand on the floor.

- Slowly twist until you feel mild tension.

- Hold for 10 seconds, then twist slightly farther until you feel slightly more tension.

- Hold this position for 10 seconds.

- Return to starting position and twist to the left side.

- Repeat sequence 2 or 3 times.

11. Chest Stretch

Chest, Shoulders, Biceps

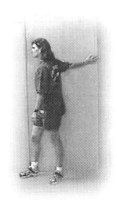

- Stand with right shoulder against a wall.

- Place right palm on the wall.

- Slowly turn your body away from the wall until you feel mild tension.

- Hold for 10 seconds, then twist slightly farther until you feel slightly more tension.

- Return to starting position and repeat sequence with left arm.

- Repeat sequence 2 or 3 times.

12. Triceps Stretch

Triceps, Posterior Deltoids

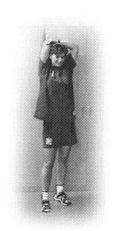

- Stand upright and extend right arm over head.
- Grab right elbow with left hand and place right hand on right shoulder blade.
- Slowly push right elbow backward until mild tension is felt.
- Hold for ten seconds, then push slightly farther until you feel slightly more tension.
- Return to starting position and repeat sequence with left arm.
- Repeat sequence 2 or 3 times.

13. Forearm Stretch

Forearms

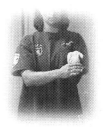

- Stand upright and grab right fingers with left hand.
- Slowly fold right wrist backwards until mild tension is felt.
- Hold for ten seconds, then push slightly farther until you feel slightly more tension.
- Repeat sequence, this time folding wrist forward.
- Return to starting position and repeat sequence with left arm.
- Repeat entire sequence 2 or 3 times.

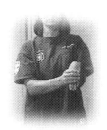

GENERAL PRINCIPLES OF EXERCISE

To maximize the results from your training program, several exercise principles should be understood. Adaptation means that the body can adjust to any overload as long as it is done in small increments. The amount of progress the body can make depends on adequate rest, consistency of workouts, adequate nutrition, and genetic makeup.

OVERLOAD

Overload, in exercise training programs, means that a training program causes the body to adapt only when the demands are greater than what the body is accustomed to doing. This does not mean that the overload is greater than your maximum, but rather that overload is generally greater than 75% of your maximal effort.

PROGRESSION

The principle of progression states that as the body adapts to the exercise program you must gradually increase the overload to continue to adapt. It is critical that all progressions are gradual and small in nature to prevent over-loading the body's ability to recover.

SPECIFICITY

Specificity of training is the principle that your body will adapt to whatever exercises you perform. This means that if you only perform bench presses, your body will not adapt to sit-ups. It may, therefore, be beneficial for you to alter your training to prepare for the Candidate Physical Ability Test.

OVER-TRAINING

Over-training addresses the body's need for adequate rest and nutrition following exercise to recuperate before the next exercise session. If recuperation is not adequate, over-training will occur. Signs of over-training include: increased injury rate, increased resting heart rate, muscle soreness that does not subside after 48 hours, apathy, insomnia, loss of appetite, lack of adaptation to exercise, and loss of strength. Over-training must be avoided.

BALANCE

When developing a strength training program, it is important to balance muscle development by including exercises that train all major muscles groups of the body. This means that if the chest is trained, the back must also be trained; similarly, if the upper body is trained, the legs must also be trained. When this principle is not followed, joints become imbalanced and injuries occur.

CARDIOPULMONARY ENDURANCE PROGRAM

Cardiopulmonary endurance is the ability of the cardiovascular and respiratory systems to deliver oxygen to working muscles. It consists of both aerobic and anaerobic energy systems.

AEROBIC FITNESS

During aerobic activities, the intensity of the exercise is low enough for the cardiopulmonary system to meet the oxygen demands of the working muscles. Aerobic activities include bicycling, hiking, swimming, climbing stairs, and running when performed at a low enough intensity.

ANAEROBIC FITNESS

During anaerobic activities, the intensity of exercise is so high that the working muscles' demands for oxygen exceed the cardiopulmonary system's ability to deliver it. Because adequate oxygen is not available, waste products accumulate. This type of intense activity can only be short in duration. An example of an anaerobic activity is sprinting.

THE CPAT TRAINING PROGRAM

The CPAT Training Program consists of two training programs. The first program is the aerobic training program and the interval program. These programs complement each other and improve your aerobic and anaerobic fitness specific to the Candidate Physical Ability Test.

AEROBIC TRAINING

The cardiopulmonary endurance program should begin at a level that is considered "moderately difficult" but not "difficult." Your intensity should not be so high that you cannot speak during the exercise. The program below consists of a series of progressive levels. As you adapt to each step, you should move up to the next level. This program should be done three to five days per week.

INTERVAL TRAINING

Interval training involves a repeated series of exercise activities interspersed with rest or relief periods. This is an excellent tool for improving both aerobic and anaerobic endurance. In this program running intervals are performed on Tuesdays and Thursdays. It is important that interval days have at least one day of slow, easy running between them. This provides the recovery necessary to prevent over-training (Table 6.1).

MUSCULAR STRENGTH/ENDURANCE PROGRAM

This is a resistance program designed to improve your total body strength and endurance. This is not a bodybuilding or a power-lifting program. It is designed to prepare you specifically for the Candidate Physical Ability Test. If you are not familiar with lifting programs, have any joint pain, or feel uncomfortable performing these exercises, you should seek the advice of a professional trainer.

This program is designed to be performed three days a week. This means that you will not be lifting four days a week. These rest days are just as important as your workout days. A critical mistake made by some applicants is over-training when preparing for the Candidate Physical Ability Test. If you feel you are over-training, refer back to the exercise principles, slow down your progression, reduce your overload, and allow for adequate rest between workouts.

This workout should follow the previously mentioned warm-up and stretching program. This program is designed to be a circuit workout. Circuit training has been proven to be a very effective and efficient way to improve muscular strength, muscular endurance, and cardiovascular endurance. Once you begin this workout, you will lift at each station for 10 repetitions and then move on to the next exercise. Rest between exercises should not exceed 30 seconds unless you are experiencing some discomfort. For safety purposes, it is recommended that you lift with a partner and spot each other when necessary.

Table 6.1 Interval Training Program

PHASE ONE

	Monday	Tuesday	Wednesday	Thursday	Friday
LEVEL 1	Run 1 mile at an easy pace being sure to be able to talk the entire time.	Run 30 seconds at a somewhat hard pace then walk for 30 seconds. Repeat this for a total of 1 mile.	Run 1 mile at an easy pace being sure to be able to talk the entire time.	Run 30 seconds at a somewhat hard pace then walk for 30 seconds. Repeat this for a total of 1 mile.	Run 1 mile at an easy pace being sure to be able to talk the entire time.
LEVEL 2	Run 1.5 miles at an easy pace being sure to be able to talk the entire time.	Run 30 seconds at a somewhat hard pace then walk for 30 seconds. Repeat this for a total of 1.5 miles.	Run 1.5 miles at an easy pace being sure to be able to talk the entire time.	Run 30 seconds at a somewhat hard pace then walk for 30 seconds. Repeat this for a total of 1.5 miles.	Run 1.5 miles at an easy pace being sure to be able to talk the entire time.
LEVEL 3	Run 2 miles at an easy pace being sure to be able to talk the entire time.	Run 60 seconds at a somewhat hard pace then walk for 60 seconds. Repeat this for a total of 2 miles.	Run 2 miles at an easy pace being sure to be able to talk the entire time.	Run 60 seconds at a somewhat hard pace then walk for 60 seconds. Repeat this for a total of 2 miles.	Run 2 miles at an easy pace being sure to be able to talk the entire time.
LEVEL 4	Run 2.5 miles at an easy pace being sure to be able to talk the entire time.	Run 60 seconds at a somewhat hard pace then walk for 60 seconds. Repeat this for a total of 2.5 miles.	Run 2.5 miles at an easy pace being sure to be able to talk the entire time.	Run 60 seconds at a somewhat hard pace then walk for 60 seconds. Repeat this for a total of 2.5 miles.	Run 2.5 miles at an easy pace being sure to be able to talk the entire time.
LEVEL 5	Run 3 miles at an easy pace being sure to be able to talk the entire time.	Run 90 seconds at a somewhat hard pace then walk for 90 seconds. Repeat this for a total of 3 miles.	Run 3 miles at an easy pace being sure to be able to talk the entire time.	Run 90 seconds at a somewhat hard pace then walk for 90 seconds. Repeat this for a total of 3 miles.	Run 3 miles at an easy pace being sure to be able to talk the entire time.

PHASE TWO

	Monday	Tuesday	Wednesday	Thursday	Friday
LEVEL 6	Run 3 miles at an easy pace being sure to be able to talk the entire time.	Run at an easy pace for 3 minutes then run stairs moderately hard for 1 minute.	Run 1.5 miles easy pace.	Run at an easy pace for 3 minutes then run stairs moderately hard for 1 minute.	Run 3 miles at an easy pace being sure to be able to talk the entire time.
LEVEL 7	Run 3 miles at an easy pace being sure to be able to talk the entire time.	Run at an easy pace for 3 minutes then run stairs moderately hard for 90 seconds.	Run 1.5 miles easy pace.	Run at an easy pace for 3 minutes then run stairs moderately hard for 90 seconds.	Run 3 miles at an easy pace being sure to be able to talk the entire time.
LEVEL 8	Run 3 miles at an easy pace being sure to be able to talk the entire time.	Run at an easy pace for 3 minutes then run stairs moderately hard for 2 minutes.	Run 1.5 miles easy pace.	Run at an easy pace for 3 minutes then run stairs moderately hard for 2 minutes.	Run 3 miles at an easy pace being sure to be able to talk the entire time.
LEVEL 9	Run 3 miles at an easy pace being sure to be able to talk the entire time.	Run at an easy pace for 3 minutes then run stairs moderately hard for 2.5 minutes.	Run 1.5 miles easy pace.	Run at an easy pace for 3 minutes then run stairs moderately hard for 2.5 minutes.	Run 3 miles at an easy pace being sure to be able to talk the entire time.
LEVEL 10	Run 3 miles at an easy pace being sure to be able to talk the entire time.	Run at an easy pace for 3 minutes then run stairs moderately hard for 3 minutes.	Run 1.5 miles easy pace.	Run at an easy pace for 3 minutes then run stairs moderately hard for 3 minutes.	Run 3 miles at an easy pace being sure to be able to talk the entire time.

GENERAL SAFETY TIPS WHILE PERFORMING RESISTANCE TRAINING

- Always lift with a partner.
- Ask for help from an expert if you don't know what you are doing.
- Progress slowly to avoid injuries.
- Never show off by attempting to lift more weight than you normally lift.
- Use proper lifting technique when lifting weight plates and dumbbells.
- Never drink alcohol or take medications that may cause drowsiness prior to lifting weights.
- Do not lift too quickly, and always control the weights.
- Always use strict form. Proper technique is more important than the amount of weight lifted.
- Keep head in a neutral position, looking straight ahead and not upward or downward.

PROGRESSION

Unless you are an experienced weightlifter, it is recommended that you begin by doing one complete cycle through this circuit. After the first week, if you are not still getting muscle soreness 24 to 48 hours after your workouts, you can progress to two cycles through the circuit. After the second week, if you are not still getting muscle soreness 24 to 48 hours after your workouts, you can progress to three cycles through the circuit. Although it is not critical, it is recommended that you follow the exercises in order. If, after progressing to the next level, you feel very sore, you many want to decrease the weights and the number of times you complete the circuit.

WEIGHT TRAINING WORKOUT

1. Seated Leg Press

Quadriceps, Hamstrings, Glutes, Calves

CPAT Events: Stair Climb, Hose Drag, Ladder Raise, Forcible Entry, Rescue, Ceiling Breach and Pull

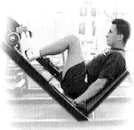

Set appropriate weight to overload above muscles, but not so heavy as to cause injury or failure.

- Place your feet flat on push platform about shoulder-width apart with toes pointed slightly outward.
- Adjust seat so knees are flexed at 90 degrees.
- Push weight up while exhaling.
- Stop just short of locking your knees.
- Keep knees in alignment with feet.
- Keep head in neutral position.

2. DB Military Press

Deltoids, Triceps, Trapezius

CPAT Events: Ladder Raise, Search, Ceiling Breach and Pull

Pick appropriate weight to overload above muscles, but not so heavy as to cause injury or failure.

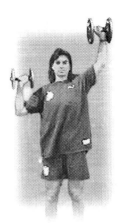

- Raise two dumbbells to height of shoulders.

- With palms facing forward, alternate pressing each dumbbell upward toward the ceiling.

- Exhale while lifting.

- Keep head in neutral position.

- Using slight leg push is acceptable.

- Repeat with other arm.

3. Lat Pull Down

Latissimus Dorsi, Rhomboids, Posterior Deltoids, Biceps

CPAT Events: Hose Drag, Ladder Extension, Forcible Entry, Rescue, Ceiling Breach and Pull

Pick appropriate weight to overload above muscles, but not so heavy as to cause injury or failure.

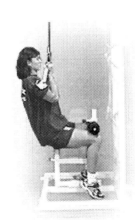

- Adjust seat and leg hold to allow full range of motion.

- Hold bar in chin-up grip with hands close together and palms toward face.

- Pull bar straight down to just below the chin.

- Exhale while pulling weight down.

- Return to starting position.

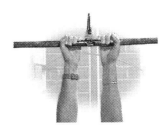

4. DB Split-Squats

Glutes, Quadriceps, Hamstrings, Calves

CPAT Events: Stair Climb, Hose Drag, Ladder Raise, Forcible Entry, Search, Rescue, Ceiling Pull and Breach

Pick a light weight (many people can start with no weights at all). Do not start with more than 10 lbs.

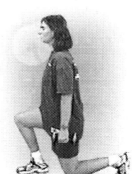

- Stand with feet together, then step backward about 26" with one foot.

- Keep back straight and arms down at side with head neutral, and slowly bend both legs.

- Lower yourself slowly until your left knee barely touches the floor.

- Forward leg should remain vertical through-out motion with knee directly over ankle. If knee tends to move forward over the toes, adjust back foot farther backward.

- Return to the starting position.

- Inhale while lowering and exhale while push-ing back up into upright position.

- Repeat with opposite leg.

5. Bench Press

Pectorals, Deltoids, Triceps

CPAT Events: Ladder Raise, Forcible Entry, Search, Ceiling Breach and Pull

Pick appropriate weight to overload above muscles, but not so heavy as to cause injury or failure.

- Lie on a bench with your feet flat on floor.

- Hold bar with arms shoulder-width apart or slightly wider.

- Lower bar to middle of chest.

- Push bar up to starting position.

- Inhale while lowering and exhale while pushing back up.

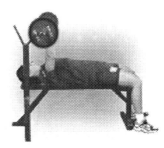

6. DB Row

Latissimus Dorsi, Rhomboids, Posterior Deltoids, Trapezius, Biceps

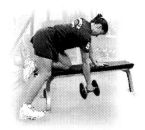

CPAT Events: Hose Pull, Ladder Extension, Forcible Entry, Rescue, Ceiling Breach and Pull

Pick appropriate weight to overload above muscles, but not so heavy as to cause injury or failure.

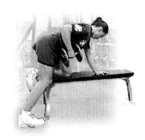

- Standing to right of bench, place left knee on bench and support upper body with left (non-lifting) arm.

- Keep head in neutral position.

- Pull DB from ground into waist area with right arm.

- Lower DB back to starting position.

- Avoid twisting at waist.

- Inhale while lowering weight and exhale while lifting weight.

- Repeat sequence on opposite side.

7. Leg Extension

Quadriceps

CPAT Events: Stair Climb, Hose Pull, Ladder Raise, Forcible Entry, Search, Rescue

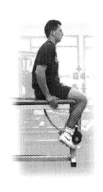

Pick appropriate weight to overload above muscles, but not so heavy as to cause injury or failure.

- Adjust machine so that backs of your knees are against the pad and back pad is supporting lower back.

- Extend knees, stopping just before the knees lock.

- Slowly lower weight to starting position.

- Exhale while pushing weight and inhale while lowering weight.

    Note: This exercise should not be performed by individuals who have undergone reconstructive knee surgery.

8. Leg Curl

Hamstrings

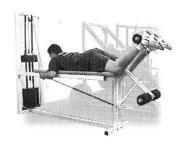

CPAT Events: Stair Climb, Hose Pull, Ladder Raise, Forcible Entry, Rescue

Pick appropriate weight to overload above muscles, but not so heavy as to cause injury or failure.

- Lie flat on the machine with top of your knees just off the pad and ankle roller situated above the heels.
- Flex the knee until ankle roller reaches the buttocks. Keep hips down and stomach in contact with pad throughout the motion.
- Slowly lower weight to starting position.
- Inhale while pulling weight up and exhale while lowering weight down.

9. DB Curl

Biceps, Forearms

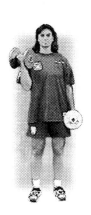

CPAT Events: Hose Drag, Ladder Extension, Forcible Entry, Rescue, Ceiling Breach and Pull

Pick appropriate weight to overload above muscles, but not so heavy as to cause injury or failure.

- Stand up with knees slightly bent.
- Begin with arms down at sides.
- Bend right elbow, bringing the dumbbell toward the right shoulder.
- Slowly lower dumbbell to starting position.
- Exhale while raising weight and inhale while lowering weight.
- Repeat sequence on opposite side.

10. Triceps Extension

Triceps

CPAT Events: Ladder Raise, Forcible Entry, Search, Ceiling Breach and Pull

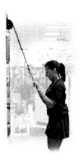

Pick appropriate weight to overload above muscles, but not so heavy as to cause injury or failure.

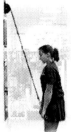

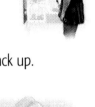

- Stand up with knees slightly bent.

- Place hands on bar about 6" apart.

- Keeping upper arms at sides, extend the elbows until arms are almost straight and bar is at mid-thigh.

- Slowly return bar to an elbow-flexed position at mid-chest level. Upper arms should remain in contact with sides. Do not allow elbows to move forward, away from body.

- Exhale while pushing bar down and inhale while returning bar back up.

11. Abdominal Curls

Abdominal Muscles

CPAT Events: All Events

- Sit on ground with knees bent at 90 degrees.

- Keeping feet flat on floor and hands at your sides, slowly curl your torso so your chin approaches your chest.

- Do not raise torso to more than a 45-degree angle off the floor.

- Slowly return to slightly above your starting position, keeping tension on abdominal muscles at all times.

- Exhale while curling up and inhale while lowering torso back down.

12. Swimmers

Erector Spinae (Lower back), Glutes

CPAT Events: All Events

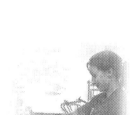

- Lie face down on ground with feet together.

- Place arms straight out in front.

- Move the right arm and left leg up at the same time.

- As you return the right arm and left leg to the starting position, move the left arm and right leg up at the same time.

- Continue alternating in a moderate cadence.

Note: Do not raise your extended leg so high as to cause discomfort in the lower back.

13. Wrist Rollers

Forearm muscles

CPAT Events: Hose Drag, Equipment Carry, Ladder Extension, Forcible Entry, Rescue, Ceiling Breach and Pull

- Stand erect.

- Set machine to "somewhat difficult" resistance.

- Grab machine with both palms facing the floor.

- Alternately roll each wrist toward the ceiling.

- Repeat with palms upward when done.

14. Hand Grippers

Forearm muscles

CPAT Events: Hose Drag, Equipment Carry, Ladder Extension, Forcible Entry, Rescue, Ceiling Breach and Pull

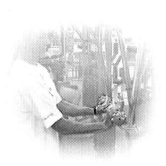

- Stand erect.

- Set machine to "somewhat difficult" resistance.

- Grab machine with both hands.

- Alternately close grip to squeeze machine.

EXERCISES WITHOUT WEIGHTS

Although it is easier to improve muscular strength and endurance with weight equipment, it is also possible to accomplish this with some simple exercises. These exercises require minimum equipment and can be done almost anywhere. Perform these exercises in a circuit. Move from one exercise to the next with minimal rest. Initially, work in the "somewhat hard" range. Do not exercise to failure. Start by going through the circuit one time and then gradually progress until you can complete this circuit three times in a row.

CALISTHENICS CIRCUIT WORKOUT

1. Chair Squats

Glutes, Quadriceps, Hamstrings

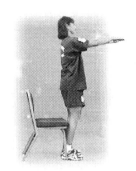

CPAT Events: Stair Climb, Hose Drag, Ladder Raise, Forcible Entry, Search, Rescue Ceiling Pull and Breach

Stand in front of a sturdy and stable chair with legs shoulder-width apart and toes pointing slightly outward.

- Hold arms out straight in front of you.

- Slowly lower your buttocks into the chair.

- As soon as you feel the slightest contact with the chair, slowly stand back up to the starting position.

- Keep your head in a neutral position.

- Inhale while lowering yourself and exhale while standing up.

2. Push Ups

Pectorals, Deltoids, Triceps, Abdominals, Low Back

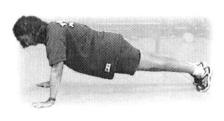

CPAT Events: Ladder Raise, Forcible Entry, Search, Ceiling Breach and Pull

Place hands on the ground at or slightly more than shoulder-width apart.

Keep feet together and back straight throughout the exercise.

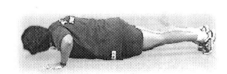

- Lower the body until the upper arms are at least parallel to the ground.

- Push yourself up to the initial position by completely straightening arms.

- Inhale while lowering and exhale while pushing.

3. Split-Squats

Glutes, Quadriceps, Hamstrings, Calves

CPAT Events: Stair Climb, Hose Drag, Ladder Raise, Forcible Entry, Search, Rescue, Ceiling Pull and Breach

Stand with feet together, then step backward about 26" with right foot.

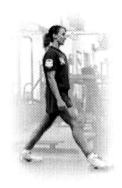

- Keep back straight and arms down at your sides with head neutral, then slowly lower the right knee straight down onto the floor.

- Inhale while lowering and exhale while pushing back up into upright position.

- Forward leg should remain vertical throughout this motion, with knee directly over ankle. If knee tends to move forward over the toes, adjust back foot farther backward.

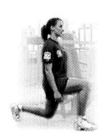

- Repeat with other leg.

4. Chin Ups

Latissimus Dorsi, Rhomboids, Posterior Deltoids, Biceps

CPAT Events: Hose Drag, Ladder Extension, Forcible Entry, Rescue, Ceiling Pull and Breach

- Grasp horizontal bar with palms facing you and hands 6" apart.

- Hang from bar with arms fully extended.

- Pull yourself upward until your chin is above the bar.

- Do not kick or swing your legs.

- Return to the starting position.

- Inhale while lowering yourself and exhale while pulling yourself up.

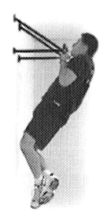

- If unable to complete three chin-ups, elevate yourself to the bar with a stool or with help from a partner, and slowly lower yourself in a slow and controlled fashion.

5. Bench Steps

Glutes, Quadriceps, Hamstrings, Calves

CPAT Events: Stair Climb, Hose Drag, Ladder Raise, Forcible Entry, Search, Rescue, Ceiling Pull and Breach

This requires good balance, so initially set the step next to a wall or use a partner for safety.

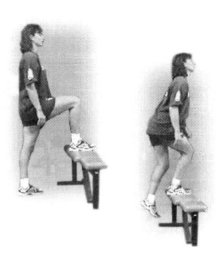

- Use a step or bench 6" to 18" high.
- Place right foot flat on the bench with the left foot flat on the floor.
- Push down with the foot on the bench and step up until both legs are straight.
- Slowly lower yourself back down to the starting position.
- Exhale while pushing up and inhale while lowering down.
- Repeat entire sequence with other leg.
- Start with a smaller step and progressively increase the height. Do not exceed 18" high.

6. Dips

Pectorals, Deltoids, Triceps

CPAT Events: Ladder Raise, Forcible Entry, Search, Ceiling Pull and Breach

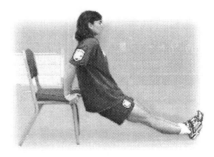

- Place hands behind you on a dip bar or chair with feet straight in front.
- Bend arms and lower body in a controlled manner until the upper arms are parallel with the floor.
- Straighten the arms to return to the starting position.
- Legs can be bent to reduce the difficulty level of the exercise.
- If unable to perform three dips, use a stool or a partner to help you up and then lower yourself slowly.
- Inhale while lowering yourself and exhale while pushing up.

7. Squat Thrusts

Pectorals, Deltoids, Triceps, Abdominals, Glutes, Quadriceps

CPAT Events: Stair Climb, Hose Pull, Ladder Raise, Forcible Entry, Search

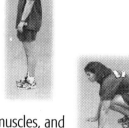

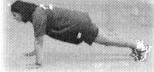

- Stand erect with feet together.

- Quickly bend knees until palms touch the floor just slightly in front of you.

- Supporting weight with arms, tighten your abdominal muscles, and throw your feet backward until you are in the push up starting position.

- Reverse sequence until you are back at the starting position. This is one repetition.

- Inhale and exhale evenly throughout the exercise.

8. Abdominal Curls

Abdominal Muscles

CPAT Events: All Events

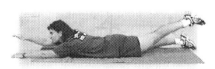

- Sit on ground with knees bent at 90 degrees.

- Keeping feet flat on floor and hands at your sides, slowly curl torso so chin approaches your chest.

- Do not raise torso to more than a 45-degree angle off the floor.

- Slowly return to slightly above your starting position, keeping tension on abdominal muscles at all times.

- Exhale while curling up and inhale while lowering torso back down.

9. Swimmers

Erector Spinae (Lower back), Glutes

CPAT Events: All Events

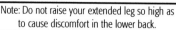

- Lie face down on ground with feet together.

- Place arms straight out in front of you.

- Move the right arm and left leg up at the same time.

- As you return the right arm and left leg to the starting position, move the left arm and right leg up at the same time.

- Continue alternating in a moderate cadence.

> Note: Do not raise your extended leg so high as to cause discomfort in the lower back.

10. Hand Grippers

Forearm muscles

CPAT Events: Hose Drag, Equipment Carry, Ladder Extension, Forcible Entry, Rescue, Ceiling Breach and Pull

- Stand erect.
- Place tennis ball in palm of hand.
- Slowly squeeze hand, compressing tennis ball.
- Repeat with other hand.

SUPPLEMENTAL TASK-SPECIFIC EXERCISE TRAINING

The supplementary exercise program presented in the following sections not only makes use of the overload principal of training but also applies the all-important principal of training specificity. Exercise training specificity means that performance improvements occur most readily when training closely resembles the specific physical activity for which improved performance is desired. When training for specific activities requiring high levels of muscular strength and muscular power (e.g., hose drag and pull from kneeling position, ladder raise and extension, sledge hammer swing, dummy drag, and ceiling breach and pull) task-specific muscular overload should accompany a general strength training program. Practice and training in the specific activity become crucial because much of the improvement in muscular strength/power performance depends upon skill learning and new muscular adaptations (i.e., coordination of specific muscle actions) required for the physical task. In most instances, training in the actual task proves most effective.

The following program provides examples for applying your general training program to actually performing CPAT tasks. As with your other preparation training, you must progressively upgrade the duration, frequency, and intensity of exercise to continually improve your performance. This will maximize your improvement in performing the CPAT.

In the beginning phase of this training, progress slowly so that you can safely learn the skill and coordination required for the movements. As you become confident in your ability to successfully complete a specific exercise task with relative ease, redirect your training energies to those activities that pose the greatest difficulty. For many people, the stair climb with full weights, forcible entry, and rescue prove the most difficult.

STAIR CLIMB
Exercise

You can readily modify aerobic training to more closely resemble the 3-minute stair climb in the CPAT by performing actual stair-stepping exercise on any conveniently located first step of a staircase, preferably at least 8 inches in height. Step at a rate that permits completion of 24 complete stepping cycles within a one-minute period. A stepping cycle consists of stepping up with one foot, then the other and down with one foot, then the other in an "up-up, down-down" rhythm. Strive to complete two stepping cycles within a five-second period.

Progression

Begin training by stepping continuously (unweighted) for five minutes. As your fitness improves, complete a second and then third five-minute exercise bout interspersed with several minutes of recovery. Once you can complete three intervals of five minutes of stepping, add weight to your torso in the form of a knapsack to which weights, sand, dirt, or rocks has been added. Continue to perform three five-minute intervals of stepping; progressively add weight to the knapsack as your fitness improves so that you can step with 50 pounds of additional weight. (This 50-pound knapsack and work gloves should be worn in training for all subsequent events of the CPAT.) In addition, carry 10-15 pounds (dumbbell, sand-filled plastic container) in each hand while stepping. The total weight carried (knapsack plus hand-held weights) should equal approximately 75 pounds.

At this stage, reduce the duration of the exercise interval to three minutes. This task-specific training not only improves aerobic fitness for continuous stepping but it also improves your leg power for stepping in the weighted condition, which represents a unique component of this CPAT item.

HOSE DRAG

Exercise

Attach 50 feet of rope to a duffel bag to which weight has been added. Tires or cement blocks can also be used for resistance. Choose an initial resistance that enables you to perform 8 to 10 repetitions (two-minute recovery between repetitions) of the exercise sequence. This generally represents an effort that you would rate as feeling "somewhat hard."

Progression

Progressively increase the resistance to 60 to 80 pounds as fitness improves. Place the rope over your shoulder and drag the resistance a distance of 75 feet. (You should run during this phase of the event.) Immediately drop to one knee and steadily and briskly pull the rope hand-over-hand to bring the resistance into your body. A parking lot, school yard, driveway, or sidewalk can be used for training on this event

EQUIPMENT CARRY

Exercise

Use two dumbbells or plastic containers filled with sand so that each weighs approximately 30 pounds. Place the weights on a shelf four feet above ground level. Remove the weights, one at a time, and place them on the ground. Then pick up the weights and carry them a distance of 40 feet out and 40 feet back and replace them on the shelf.

Progression

If the initial weight feels too heavy, choose a lighter weight for your initial practice. Continue to practice this test item until it can be performed with 30 pounds with relative ease.

LADDER RAISE AND EXTENSION

Exercise

Ladder Raise. The ideal training for this task requires an actual 12-foot aluminum extension ladder. If this size ladder is unavailable, you can use a single ladder or smaller extension ladder to practice the skill required for raising the ladder. Practice of the ladder raise sequence requires the assistance of two adults to "foot" the ladder at its base to prevent it form sliding forward and/or falling during the raise. In practicing this component (as described in the test directions) it is important to initially move slowly so as to develop the skill and confidence to safely complete the required movements. Be sure to use each rung when raising the ladder to develop the coordination and timing necessary on the CPAT.

Exercise

Ladder Extension. Task-specific training of the muscles required in the ladder extension can be provided by attaching a rope to a weighted duffel bag or knapsack. Place the rope over a tree branch (or horizontal bar support above a row of playground swings) eight to ten feet above the ground. With hand-over-hand movements, steadily raise the bag to the top of the branch or bar and then slowly lower it to the ground.

Progression

Start with a weight that you would rate as feeling "somewhat hard," and perform eight to ten repetitions of the movement. Rest two minutes and repeat the exercise-rest sequence two more times. As your strength improves, progressively add more resistance until you can exercise with 40 to 50 pounds of weight.

FORCIBLE ENTRY

Exercise

Borrow or purchase a 10-pound sledgehammer. Wrap padding around a large tree or vertical pole at a level of 39 inches above the ground with a circular target in the center. Stand sideways and swing the sledgehammer in a level manner so the head strikes the center of the target area. Focus on using your legs and hips to initiate the swinging motion.

Progression

The initial phase of this task-specific training should focus on learning the coordinated movement of your arms and legs to accurately hit the target. Repeat the swing 15 times and rest for two minutes. Repeat this exercise-rest sequence twice again. Strive to increase the velocity (power) of each swing without sacrificing accuracy as your comfort level and skill on this test item improve.

SEARCH

Exercise

Practice crawling on hands and knees (wearing sweat pants and/or kneepads) at least 70 feet while making several right angle turns during the crawl. For the major portion of the crawl, keep low enough so as not to contact an object three feet above the ground. Periodically, drop your stomach and crawl ten feet along the ground.

Progression

Once you are comfortable crawling as above repeat the sequence with a knapsack on. Gradually increase the weight within the knapsack until it equals 50 pounds.

RESCUE
Exercise

Attach a short handle to a duffel bag to which rocks, sand, or other appropriate weight can be progressively added. Start with a weight that feels "somewhat heavy." You can grasp the handle with (a) one hand and drag the "victim" in a cross-over, side-stepping manner, or (b) two hands while facing the "victim" and moving directly backward while taking short, rapid stagger steps. Drag the weight 35 to 50 feet in one direction turn around and drag it back to the starting point. Complete eight to ten repetitions of this task with a two-minute rest interval between each trial.

Progression

Gradually increase the resistance until you can successfully complete four repetitions (with rest interval) with 165 pounds.

CEILING BREACH AND PULL
Exercise

Ceiling Breach. Tie a rope to a dumbbell or weighted knapsack placed between your legs, shoulder-width apart. Grasp the rope, arms slightly away from the body with one hand at upper-thigh level and the other hand at chest level. Lift upward and out from the body in an action that simulates thrusting a pole through an overhead ceiling. Use a resistance that feels "somewhat hard," yet enables you to complete three sets of eight repetitions with two minutes of rest between sets.

Progression

Continually add weight as strength improves. Practice coordinating upward arm movements with an upward extension of the legs to provide a more powerful thrusting action.

Exercise

Ceiling Pull. The training set-up for this simulation is the same as that used in training for the ladder extension. However, unlike the hand-over-hand movement that is required for the ladder extension, the ceiling pull requires exerting power in single, repeated downward thrusts. Grasp the rope attached to the weighted knapsack or duffel bag with hands spaced about one-foot apart and the bottom hand at chin level. With a powerful movement, simultaneously pull arms down and lower your body to raise weight several feet above the ground. Repeat eight to 10 consecutive repetitions of the movement with a resistance that feels "somewhat hard." Complete three sets with a two-minute recovery interval interspersed.

Progression

Progressively add resistance as fitness improves. As your fitness improves you should begin to link the various test components. For example, immediately upon finishing the stair climb move directly to the hose drag and then to the equipment carry. Eventually you will be able to simulate all of the task components in the CPAT in a continuous exercise sequence.

IAFF/IAFC CANDIDATE PHYSICAL ABILITY TEST
Preparation Guide Strength Training Log
[No Weights]

Name_____

Exercise	Date															
1 Chair Squats	Weight	X	X	X	X	X	X	X	X	X	X	X	X	X	X	X
	Reps	20														
2 Push Ups	Weight	X	X	X	X	X	X	X	X	X	X	X	X	X	X	X
	Reps															
3 Split Squats	Weight	X	X	X	X	X	X	X	X	X	X	X	X	X	X	X
	Reps	10														
4 Chin Ups	Weight	X	X	X	X	X	X	X	X	X	X	X	X	X	X	X
	Reps															
5 Bench Steps	Weight	X	X	X	X	X	X	X	X	X	X	X	X	X	X	X
	Reps	10														
6 Dips	Weight	X	X	X	X	X	X	X	X	X	X	X	X	X	X	X
	Reps															
7 Squat Thrusts	Weight	X	X	X	X	X	X	X	X	X	X	X	X	X	X	X
	Reps	10														
8 Abdominal Curls	Weight	X	X	X	X	X	X	X	X	X	X	X	X	X	X	X
	Reps	20														
9 Swimmers	Weight	X	X	X	X	X	X	X	X	X	X	X	X	X	X	X
	Reps	15														
10 Hand Grippers	Weight	Tennis Ball	Tennis Ball	Tennis Ball	Tennis Ball	Tennis Ball	Tennis Ball	Tennis Ball	Tennis Ball	Tennis Ball	Tennis Ball	Tennis Ball	Tennis Ball	Tennis Ball	Tennis Ball	Tennis Ball
	Reps	15														

IAFF/IAFC CANDIDATE PHYSICAL ABILITY TEST
Preparation Guide Strength Training Log

Name_____

	Exercise	Date	Weight	Reps
1	Seated Leg Press			20
2	DB Military Press			10
3	Lat Pulldown Front			10
4	DB Single Leg Squat			10
5	Bench Press			10
6	Seated Row			10
7	Leg Extension			10
8	Leg Curl			10
9	DB Bicep Curl			10
10	Tricep Extensions			10
11	Abdominal Curls			20
12	Swimmers			15
13	Wrist Rollers			10
14	Hand Grippers			10

STRENGTH
TRAINING

Fire fighting is a very strenuous job that requires high levels of muscular strength and endurance in order to perform successfully and avoid injuries. Designing strength training programs is one of the primary duties of PFTs. This chapter reviews the key components of strength training as it pertains to the fire service.

DEFINITIONS

Several key strength training terms are often used incorrectly, leading to confusion and misinformation. Definitions of these key terms are given below.

Muscular Strength – the ability to exert a maximal force at a given speed in a single voluntary contraction

Muscular Endurance – the ability to exert a submaximal force for multiple voluntary contractions or one extended contraction

Power – force multiplied by velocity as shown by the following formula:
Power = F x (D/T) = F x V if F= force, D= distance, T=time, V=velocity
Since work equals force times distance, power can also be expressed as work divided by time.

Volume – the total amount of weight lifted in a workout session
Volume = weight lifted x reps x sets

Skill – the ability to perform complex motor movements efficiently

CHAPTER

7

KEY STRENGTH FACTORS

There are several key factors that affect an individual's ability to increase strength. In order to help your clients set realistic goals, it is important to know how these factors affect the response to a strength training program. The key factors influencing an individual's strength are sex, age, heredity, and training factors.

SEX

Prior to puberty there are very few differences between boys and girls relative to muscular strength. Although pre-adolescent boys and girls can significantly improve their strength by resistance training, these gains come predominantly from increased ability to recruit muscle fibers. During puberty, girls increase their estrogen production and boys increase their testosterone production. This leads to an increase in fat deposition in females and an increase in lean body mass and bone formation in males.

In general, women are weaker than men in absolute strength because they have less lean body mass. But, when compared using lean body mass or cross-sectional area of muscle, there is no difference in strength between men and women. There is very little difference between the sexes in response to resistance training. Initial responses are identical. Longitudinal responses appear to favor men, probably due mostly to the difference in testosterone levels. It should be noted that there are just as drastic strength differences among males as there is between males and females.

Since the physiological characteristics of muscle in both sexes are the same, there is no reason why resistance training programs for women need to be drastically different from those for men. In fact, because the muscle groups involved in fire fighting are obviously the same for men and women, resistance training programs should be designed to improve the performance of the muscles needed for successful performance, regardless of sex.

AGE

As previously stated, age has a significant effect on hormonal responses. During puberty, testosterone levels increase in males. Advancing age is associated with a loss of muscle mass (specifically fast-twitch fiber atrophy), which results in a loss of strength and power. While the rate of decline is appreciably lower in those who continue to perform regular resistance exercise, there is still a natural decline. Probably the greatest impact is the effect of age on recovery. As age advances, the length of time required between resistance exercise bouts increases to allow for adequate recovery.

HEREDITY

Anyone who participates in a properly designed resistance training program will improve his or her strength; however, heredity plays a substantial role in a person's strength potential. Heredity influences a person's somatotype (general body type), which is classified as mesomorph (muscular), ectomorph (thin), or endomorph (rotund).

Certain genetic factors have an impact on strength potential. These factors include muscle density, muscle attachments (mechanical advantages), limb length (levers), muscle fiber composition, and testosterone levels.

TRAINING FACTORS

Unlike the previously listed factors, which impact a person's ultimate strength potential, the greatest and most controllable factors are training factors. These training factors are the core of the design of any strength training program, and include frequency of training, resistance loads, progression of overload, duration of training, volume of training, recovery, nutrition, and specificity of training.

BENEFITS OF STRENGTH TRAINING

There are numerous benefits to strength training, including improved ability to perform fire fighting tasks as well as enhanced physical and mental health. PFTs should therefore include strength training in every exercise program. Some of the benefits of strength training are described below.

- Increased muscular strength and endurance

  The most obvious benefit of resistance training is improvement in muscular strength and endurance. It is generally accepted by exercise professionals that by gradually increasing the amount of resistance lifted, muscular strength will be improved. During the initial few months of a training program, untrained men and women can gain 2 to 4 pounds of muscle and gain 40 to 60% more strength. Similarly, by gradually overloading the muscle's ability to resist fatigue or recuperate, muscular endurance will be improved.

- Improved body composition

  Resistance exercise can increase lean-body mass and therefore reduce the percentage of body fat. The degree of these changes depends on intensity of the resistance training, caloric intake, overall caloric expenditure, and adherence to a long-term balanced exercise program.

- Increased bone density

  Resistance exercise increases the density of connective tissues supporting the targeted muscles. This adaptation has a positive effect on bone density. Studies have demonstrated a significant positive correlation between bone mineral density and the strength and mass of the attached musculature (Pocock et al., 1989).

- Improved ability to perform activities of daily living

  For the civilian public many activities of daily living (i.e., carrying groceries, vacuuming, moving furniture) require muscular strength and endurance. For fire fighters, with equipment in excess of 75 pounds, the activities of daily living (i.e., forcible entry, pulling hose, raising ladders) require above average levels of muscular strength and endurance.

- Improved metabolism

  Strength training has a dual effect on energy metabolism. It produces a moderate increase in metabolic rate during a workout and a very mild increase in metabolic rate throughout the day due to the fact that the added muscle requires a constant supply of energy to support its cellular functions. Strength training also helps counteract the loss of lean muscle mass often associated with dieting that leads to significant weight loss. For these reasons, strength training is an important component of an effective weight management program.

- Lower risk of injury

  Sprains and strains, the most common injuries among fire fighters, are caused when external forces exceed the muscles' or joints' abilities to resist those forces. By increasing muscular strength, the number and severity of injuries can be reduced in fire fighters. It is estimated that up to 80% of low-back problems are preventable by strengthening the muscles of the low-back.

- Improved cardiac profile

  While resistance training alone may not improve maximal oxygen consumption, it has been shown to improve the ability of the heart, lungs, and circulatory system to function under conditions of high pressure and force production. Muscles performing resistance training require significantly increased blood supplies and therefore place demands on these systems. As the muscles being trained adapt to this overload, so will the systems that support those muscles. This in turn may contribute to decreased resting blood pressure, a reduced blood pressure response to resistance-type work or exercise, and improved blood lipid profiles.

- Improved self-esteem

  One of the most powerful benefits of resistance training is improved self-esteem, which can permeate all aspects of a fire fighter's life. When job duties are easier to perform, body composition is enhanced, healthy workout habits are maintained, and fitness is improved, a fire fighter's self-esteem will undoubtedly improve.

STRENGTH TRAINING VARIABLES

Several training variables must be managed by the PFT when designing resistance training programs. When these variables are not properly managed, the benefits of the program will be reduced, overtraining may occur, and injuries may result. The critical training variables are frequency, intensity, time, and type.

FREQUENCY

Frequency of resistance training refers to how often your fire fighters workout. More specifically, frequency refers to how often each individual body part will be trained, and depends on several factors:

- ☑ Time available – One of the primary factors that affect the design of the resistance program and the frequency of training is how many days per week the fire fighter has available to train.

- ☑ Goals of the fire fighter – The goals of the fire fighter dictate everything, but especially the frequency of training. PFTs must determine whether the fire fighter's goal is maintenance, improvement, performance, or rehabilitation.

- ☑ Intensity of training – As training intensity is increased, training frequency must be decreased to avoid overtraining.

- ☑ State of recovery – PFTs must constantly assess fire fighters for overtraining. If any signs or symptoms of overtraining develop, the frequency of training may need to be adjusted.

INTENSITY

Intensity of resistance training can be expressed in weight, level of resistance, RPE, or percent of maximal ability, among others. Intensity must be high enough to provide an overload for training adaptations to occur. Factors affecting the intensity of training include the following:

- ☑ Time available – As time available decreases, one method of ensuring adequate overload is by increasing training intensity.

- ☑ Goals of the fire fighter – The goals of the fire fighter help determine the intensity of training. PFTs must determine if each fire fighter's goal is maintenance, improvement, performance, or rehabilitation. As a fire fighter approaches their genetic and training capabilities, high intensities may be required to achieve even small amounts of improvement. In these cases, give close supervision and attention to overtraining.

- ☑ Frequency of training – As training frequency is increased, intensity must be lowered to avoid overtraining.

☑ State of recovery – PFTs must constantly assess fire fighters for overtraining. If any signs or symptoms of overtraining develop, the intensity of training may need to be reduced.

☑ Periodization – When using the periodization model of training, the phase of training (endurance/hypertrophy, strength, strength/power, competition) dictates the intensity of training.

TIME (DURATION)

Exercise duration is most commonly referred to as the length of workout time. While this may apply accurately for aerobic endurance exercise training, it can be vague and non-descriptive for resistance training. In this section, duration refers to total workout time. Like all aspects of resistance training, duration must progress slowly to avoid overtraining. Similarly, as intensity increases, duration must decrease. One advantage of increasing the frequency of training by splitting up the routine is that it can reduce the duration and therefore allow for an increase in intensity. The factors affecting the duration of a strength training program include the following:

☑ Goals – As always, the goals of the fire fighter are the focus of the design of any program. If the fire fighter has certain time limits, design a program that fits within them. When time limits are ignored, fire fighters may become frustrated and stop adhering to their program.

☑ Type of workout – If the fire fighter's goal is strength improvement, more rest is required between sets and exercises, and the overall duration is extended. Similarly, if the fire fighter's goal is muscular endurance, rests between sets and exercises are kept to a minimum.

☑ State of recovery – Decrease the duration of the workout when a fire fighter is overtrained. As the purpose of the workout changes from overload to active recovery, duration should also be shortened.

☑ Level of training – Training session duration is limited by the fire fighter's ability to maintain concentration and technique throughout the entire session. Fire fighters can increase this ability by progressively increasing the strength session duration. When strength sessions exceed one hour, PFTs should consider breaking up sessions into multiple shorter sessions.

TYPE (SPECIFICITY)

Doing appropriate exercise is critical to achieving each fire fighter's goals and preventing injuries. When the same exercises are used without variation, the result is increased muscle strength in only one plane or movement. This, in turn, can contribute to injuries and limit the transfer of strength to actual fire fighting tasks. Therefore, exercises should be selected with functionality, balance, and variety in mind. The factors affecting the type of exercises selected include the following:

☑ Goals of the fire fighter – PFTs must combine each fire fighter's goals with the demands of the job when choosing exercises.

☑ Lifting experience – The fire fighter's inexperience may limit the exercise selection. Some exercises require more coordination and balance, and PFTs may have to work progressively to more advanced lifts.

☑ Injuries – A fire fighter's previous and current injuries can affect exercise selection in three ways. First, injuries may limit the ability to perform certain exercises. These exercises should be identified and avoided to prevent further injury. Second, injuries may limit the range of motion of certain exercises. These exercises may be performed, but only within a pain-free, safe range of motion. Finally, injuries may identify imbalances or weaknesses that should be addressed. Many injuries result from weakness of a specific joint. Some injuries actually result from an anterior/posterior or medial/lateral muscle imbalance, which can lead to lack of stabilization and subsequent injury.

☑ Available equipment – Equipment available to the fire fighter affects exercise selection. PFTs should use insight and imagination to design a variety of exercises using available equipment. In addition, excellent exercise programs can be designed using body weight and a few inexpensive adjuncts (e.g., thera-balls, resistance bands, balance boards, and chairs).

VOLUME OF TRAINING

Volume of training refers to the total load lifted during a session. It is a concept that encompasses all of the training variables.

Weight lifted x Repetitions x Sets = Training Volume

Specific training volumes are required to achieve specific individual goals. A typical progression in training volume starts with increasing the number of sets per exercise, then increasing exercises per body part, and finally increasing resistance per set. The training volume concept makes it clear that any increase in repetitions per exercise, sets per exercise, exercises per body part, or weight lifted per exercise must progress slowly to prevent overtraining.

FUNCTIONAL TRAINING

Functional training is training the body in such a way that the strength or endurance gained directly benefits the execution of ADLs and movements associated with sports or occupations. It is a relatively new trend in strength training, which developed from a generation of strength trainers who questioned conventional methods and looked for more practical and innovative ways to implement the specificity-of-training principle.

While traditional strength training focuses on training specific muscle groups and muscles, functional strength training focuses more on the movement itself. These movements recruit various muscle groups from multiple joints in varying types of contractions (i.e., isometric, isotonic, concentric, eccentric) in a similar fashion to their actual applied use. With functional training, the muscles are trained specifically in the range of motion and context in which they will be recruited in the actual movement.

Functional training increases balance around joints and helps prevent injuries by stimulating stabilizing muscles. Most functional training focuses on core stabilizers (i.e., abdominal muscle group, back extensor muscle group), which stabilize all movement. Functional training has been extremely successful in athletic injury rehabilitation and is showing similar success in training competitive athletes. Similarly, functional training has been instrumental in implementation of work capacity evaluations and work hardening programs for fire fighters. These programs help prepare fire fighters to perform actual tasks required by the job.

The following process in developing a strength training program also applies to functional training. The key to improving the functional application of any exercise or program is in being able to apply functional training principles creatively.

DESIGNING A STRENGTH TRAINING PROGRAM

When developing any resistance training program it is important that the current training supports all future training. This approach is built into the periodization models of training that are covered later in this section. For successful strength training, target muscles and their associated tendons must be able to withstand the volume of training necessary to handle heavy loads. Similarly, target muscles and corresponding tendons must be adequately strengthened before they can tolerate power and speed training. Resistance training programs should begin by developing muscular endurance and hypertrophy, progress to muscular strength, and then, if applicable, progress to power and speed.

The systematic approach presented in Table 7.1 simplifies the process of developing strength training programs and ensures safe and effective training. These steps are discussed in detail in this section.

Table 7.1 Steps to Designing a Strength Training Program

---

1 Perform a needs analysis:
    a. help the fire fighter develop realistic goals
    b. perform a health risk assessment
    c. assess the fire fighter's current level of fitness and lifting experience
    d. determine the fire fighter's time restraints
2. Determine the general program design (e.g., total body vs. split workout)
3. Select the type of equipment
4. Select the number of exercises
	5. Select the exercises
	6. Select the number of sets per exercise
	7. Develop the exercise order
	8. Select the number of repetitions per set
	9. Determine the load/resistance for each set and exercise
	10. Determine the progression schedule
	11. Set a date to assess progress and needs and then to update the program

STEP ONE: PERFORMING A NEEDS ANALYSIS

Needs analysis drives the program design process and determines the task-specific needs of both the individual and the activity or sport. PFTs analyze physiological, biomechanical, and nutritional needs to design a program. The program design must be realistic and integrated with the goals of the fire department and the fire fighter's current fitness level, strength training experience, and time considerations.

STEP TWO: CHOOSING THE GENERAL PROGRAM DESIGN

The two general program designs are the total-body routine and the split-body routine. In the total-body routine, all the major muscle groups are trained on the same day. This workout is usually performed two to three times per week with one to three days of rest between workouts. The total-body routine is most commonly used with fire fighters who have limited time and whose goals are general strength and muscular endurance.

In the split-body routine different muscle groups are trained on different days. The most common routine trains the lower body one day, the upper body the next day, followed by a day of rest. Another routine trains the back/trapezius/biceps on one day, the legs on the next day, the chest/shoulders/triceps on the third day, followed by a rest day. A third routine trains the chest/back on one day, the legs on the next day, the shoulders/arms on the third day, followed by a rest day. A final common split routine is to train the legs on one day, the chest on the next day, the back on the third day, the shoulders on the fourth day, the arms on the fifth day, followed by a rest day. These split routines are designed for intermediate and advanced lifters and are used for those interested in bodybuilding.

STEP THREE: SELECTING THE TYPE OF EQUIPMENT

The availability and type of equipment are key factors of program design. Resistance machines typically are safer and easier to use for beginners. Free weights offer more variety, but require higher levels of skill and coordination. Other types of resistance equipment, such as stability balls, medicine balls, balance boards, and resistance bands, can also be very effective in improving strength and endurance. Use a variety of equipment and exercises to minimize boredom, and teach how to perform exercises safely and independently for each piece of equipment.

STEP FOUR: SELECTING THE NUMBER OF EXERCISES

The number of selected exercises directly affects volume of training. In the beginning stages of a program, one exercise per major muscle group is usually sufficient. Gradually increase to two or more exercises per major muscle group, depending on the program design, time restrictions, and rest periods between workouts.

STEP FIVE: SELECTING THE EXERCISES

Exercise selection depends on the needs analysis and the equipment available. Ultimately, the exercises must be within the fire fighter's experience and specific to needs and goals. PFTs must select exercises that balance each joint with adequate stimulation of both agonistic and antagonistic muscle groups.

Exercises can be classified as either core or supplemental depending on the muscle groups involved and the type of action performed. Core exercises are functional in nature, involve multiple joints, and recruit large muscle groups (i.e., legs, back, chest, abdominals, and gluteals). These types of exercises are the foundation of most performance-related programs that require functional strength and muscular power. Supplemental exercises usually involve only one primary joint, recruit smaller muscle groups, and have less direct functional applications. These exercises are commonly utilized in sport-specific and body building programs.

STEP SIX: SELECTING THE NUMBER OF SETS OF EACH EXERCISE

The number of sets performed of each exercise is a significant variable in the volume of training. Studies have suggested that higher volumes (i.e., more than one set) are necessary to promote further gains in strength, especially for intermediate and advanced resistance trained athletes (Baechle & Groves, 1998; Jones, 1971; Luthi et al., 1986; Stone & O'Bryant, 1987; Westcott, 1986).

The needs analysis influences how many sets of each exercise should be performed. Fire fighters with little experience should initially perform one set per exercise. As they adapt to the overload, the number of sets can be gradually increased to three sets per exercise. If the goal of the fire fighter is to increase muscular endurance, then three sets of high repetitions with one to two minutes of rest between sets should be performed. If the goal is maximal muscular strength or muscular power, then five sets of low repetitions with approximately three minutes of rest between sets should be performed. If the goal is muscular size, then four to six sets of moderate repetitions with 30 to 60 seconds of rest between sets should be performed.

STEP SEVEN: DEVELOPING THE EXERCISE ORDER

The sequence of exercises affects the fire fighter's performance on all subsequent exercises. Power exercises, such as the power clean, should be performed early in the workout while the fire fighter is not fatigued. If power exercises are not included, then multi-joint or core exercises should be performed before single-joint or assistance exercises. This allows the body to warm up by using larger muscle groups first, and prevents fatigue from impacting exercise technique in more complex lifts.

Grouping exercises into antagonistic movements or into upper/lower body movements can provide recovery between exercises and decrease the duration of the workout. These types of workouts (i.e., superset, circuit training) can improve cardiorespiratory endurance, muscular endurance, and muscular strength (Gettman & Pollock, 1981). Such workouts can also be designed to simulate actual job functions and maximize the crossover benefits of training, ultimately improving job performance. Examples of these types of resistance exercise programs can be found later in this section.

STEP EIGHT: SELECTING THE NUMBER OF REPETITIONS

The number of repetitions per set is a significant variable of training volume and so must be linked to the needs analysis and goals of the fire fighter. Increases in repetitions should be made in small, measured doses.

Most research involving the general public recommends 8 to 12 repetitions per set. Fire fighters wishing to improve their muscular endurance should perform 15 or more repetitions per set. Fire fighters wishing to improve their muscular strength should perform six or less repetitions per set with increased loads. Fire fighters wishing to train specifically for power should perform three to five repetitions per set of any explosive exercises. Finally, fire fighters wishing to improve muscular size should perform 6 to 12 repetitions per set to muscle failure.

STEP NINE: DETERMINING THE LOAD/RESISTANCE

The load chosen for each set is often considered the most critical variable in training volume. Increasing the load too quickly or choosing too great an initial load may lead to overtraining and injury. Selection of a safe yet stimulating training load is essential.

There are several methods of determining the proper training load. Most advocate evaluating current strength to determine one repetition maximum (1RM), then designing a strength program based on a percentage of a 1RM. Unfortunately, there are several shortcomings to this approach:

- It can be dangerous to perform maximal strength testing with inexperienced lifters.
- It assumes that the relationship between load and repetitions is linear and truly accurate.
- It requires testing of every muscle group or movement the trainer is going to train in the workout program.

In most situations, there is no reason to test the actual 1RM with fire fighters. Testing with a 10RM load (and then estimating or predicting the 1RM) is appropriate. Table 7.2 estimates a fire fighter's 1RM after testing strength within the 1-to-15 repetition range. Guidelines for strength testing for program design include the following:

- Provide a warm-up with light resistance
- Provide at least a one-minute interval between sets (should need no more than two to three sets)
- Estimate the starting load based upon the fire fighter's past experience and strength
- Gradually increase the load
- Never increase the load to a level where the fire fighter no longer lifts with proper technique

Table 7.2 Percent of the 1RM and Repetitions Allowed

%1RM	Number of Repetitions Allowed
100	1
95	2
93	3
90	4
87	5
85	6
83	7
80	8
77	9
75	10
70	11
67	12
65	15

Adapted, by permission, from T.R. Baechle, R.W. Earle, and D. Wathen, 2000, "Resistance training" in *Essentials of Strength Training and Conditioning*, 2nd ed., NSCA, edited by T.R. Baechle & R.W. Earle (Champaign, IL: Human Kinetics), 410-411.

Some fire fighters are intimidated by the idea of extensive pre-programming testing. They may perceive this step as probing, time consuming, and even intrusive. This can be a barrier to motivating them to participate in strength training programs. Another acceptable method is omitting strength testing. Instead, estimate an easy starting weight based upon the fire fighter's previous experience and lifting loads. Provided that the weight is significantly less than the fire fighter's maximum strength capacity, there is room for slow and gradual progression while minimizing the risk of overtraining. This method still provides a baseline for future comparisons.

STEP TEN: DETERMINING THE PROGRESSION SCHEDULE

As fire fighters adapt to their training programs, PFTs must consider the following questions prior to increasing the resistance for future workouts:

- Is the fire fighter adequately recovering between workouts?

- Is it appropriate to increase the number of sets while maintaining the same load?

- Is it appropriate to add an additional exercise rather than increase the load?

- Does the fire fighter use proper technique and is he or she capable of increasing the load without affecting technique?

- Is an increase in resistance consistent with the fire fighter's goals (i.e., strength or hypertrophy rather than endurance or maintenance)?

Once the PFT has answered "yes" to these questions, a conservative increase in load should be made to avoid injury or overtraining syndrome. One acceptable guideline is called the 2-for-2 rule. If the fire fighter can perform two more repetitions than assigned in the last set for two or more workouts, then it is time to slightly increase the load for the next workout (Baechle & Groves, 1998).

STEP ELEVEN: FOLLOW UP

After designing each strength training program, PFTs should follow up on the fire fighter's progress, by appointment if necessary. In the absence of this follow-up, fire fighters may freelance and change their programs, often for the worse. Scheduled follow-ups are both for developing trainer/client relationship and for improving program safety and effectiveness. Follow-up appointments every three to six weeks are usually adequate, but more frequent follow-ups may be necessary early in the program.

DESIGN FOR SUCCESS

SET REALISTIC GOALS

Setting reasonable and achievable goals helps increase the potential for realizing success, while setting unattainable goals often leads to frustration and negatively affects motivation.

DO NOT MEASURE TOO FREQUENTLY

Periodic exercise assessments are necessary and recommended, but testing too frequently may be counterproductive. The initial benefits and gains, such as weekly body weight changes, may not readily appear or may appear insignificant and weaken motivation. Follow-up testing should occur no sooner than six weeks after starting a program.

SET UP A REWARD SYSTEM

Some fire fighters are motivated by external reward systems. In these cases, rewards for progress, participation, or both may be primary motivational tools. With fire fighters who are more intrinsically motivated, verbal praise and subtle recognition of progress may work best.

AVOID PAIN

Any workout that is painful will eventually be avoided. Remember that pain is a safety mechanism that inhibits certain behaviors. While any workout may produce temporary discomfort, adherence to any program will be diminished if pain is experienced on a regular basis.

KEEP IT SIMPLE

Legend tells the story of Milo who began his training by lifting a young bull. As the bull grew heavier Milo grew stronger. This story highlights the benefits of progressive resistance and also demonstrates how simple a workout can be. Workouts can be as simple or complex as you want to make them. Making a resistance training program unduly complex can confuse and ultimately destroy fire fighter motivation. As a general rule, keep workouts as simple as possible.

THE PROPER TIME

The time of day is a critical factor for many fire fighters in adherence to their exercise programs. Exercising in the beginning of the day significantly improves adherence for most fire fighters. As the day progresses and other duties accumulate, fatigue sets in, excuses build, and it is much more likely that exercise will be sacrificed. PFTs should recommend to most fire fighters that they try to perform their workouts first thing in the day.

SAMPLE STRENGTH TRAINING WORKOUTS

SAMPLE SPLIT-ROUTINE WORKOUT #1

Split-routine workouts are designed for the fire fighter who has approximately one hour, four times per week for strength training. They are designed to balance upper- and lower-body and anterior and posterior muscle groups. The sets, repetitions, weights, days, and exercises can be changed to meet specific needs. Cardiovascular and flexibility exercises are also recommended for a total program.

FOUR-DAY SPLIT ROUTINE • *Upper Body/Lower Body*
Tuesday and Friday

Exercise	Weight	Repetitions	Sets
Squats	80% 1RM	8-10	3
Leg Press	80% 1RM	8-10	3
Leg Extension	80% 1RM	8-10	3
Leg Curl	80% 1RM	8-10	3
Calf Raises	80% 1 RM	8-10	3

Monday and Thursday

Exercise	Weight	Repetitions	Sets
Flat Bench Barbell	80% 1RM	8-10	3
Seated Row	80% 1RM	8-10	3
Incline Bench	80% 1RM	8-10	3
V-Bar Pulldowns	80% 1RM	8-10	3
DB Lateral Raises	80% 1RM	8-10	3
EZ-curl-bar Curls	80% 1RM	8-10	3
Standing Tricep Extensions	80% 1RM	8-10	3
Abdominal Crunches	Bodyweight	25	3

SAMPLE SPLIT-ROUTINE WORKOUT #2

This routine is designed for fire fighters with limited time. The sets, repetitions, weights, days, and exercises can be changed to meet specific needs. Cardiovascular and flexibility exercises are also recommended for a total program.

FIVE-DAY SPLIT ROUTINE • *One Body Part/Day*

Monday (Legs)

Exercise	Weight	Repetitions	Sets
Squats	75% 1RM	8 to 12	3
Single-leg Leg Press	75% 1RM	8 to 12	3
Leg Extension	75% 1RM	8 to 12	3
Leg Curl	75% 1RM	8 to 12	3
Calf Raises	75% 1RM	8 to 12	3

Tuesday (Chest)

Exercise	Weight	Repetitions	Sets
Flat Bench Barbell	75% 1RM	8 to 12	3
DB Incline Bench	75% 1RM	8 to 12	3
Cable Crossovers	75% 1RM	8 to 12	3
Pec Deck	75% 1RM	8 to 12	3

Wednesday (Back)

Exercise	Weight	Repetitions	Sets
Chin Ups	Bodyweight	8 to 12	3
Seated Row	75% 1RM	8 to 12	3
Lat Pull Down (wide grip)	75% 1RM	8 to 12	3
DB Row	75% 1RM	8 to 12	3
Hyperextensions	Bodyweight	8 to 12	3

Thursday (Shoulders)

Exercise	Weight	Repetitions	Sets
Barbell Military Press	75% 1RM	8 to 12	3
DB Frontal Raises	75% 1RM	8 to 12	3
Upright Rows	75% 1RM	8 to 12	3
Cable Back Flyes	75% 1RM	8 to 12	3

Friday (Arms)

Exercise	Weight	Repetitions	Sets
Curl-Bar Curls	75% 1RM	8 to 12	3
Seated DB Curls	75% 1RM	8 to 12	3
Standing Tricep Pressdowns	75% 1RM	8 to 12	3
Tricep Kickbacks	75% 1RM	8 to 12	3
Seated Palm-Up Wrist Curls	75% 1RM	8 to 12	3
Seated Reverse Wrist Curls	75% 1RM	8 to 12	3

SUPERSET AND COMPOUND SET WORKOUTS

Superset and compound set workouts pair exercises with little or no rest between them. Although these two terms are often used interchangeably, they are quite different.

A superset design uses two successive exercises that stress antagonistic muscle groups. An example is a bench press immediately followed by a seated row. While one muscle group is being stressed, the opposite muscle group is being rested. This method increases the cardiorespiratory response by increasing overall blood lactate levels and significantly reduces the duration of the workout. This is an excellent way for fire fighters to train since it is similar to performing actual fire fighting tasks.

A compound set design uses two successive exercises. Unlike a superset design, a compound set stresses agonistic muscle groups. An example is performing a bench press immediately followed by a dumbbell chest fly. Both of these exercises stress the chest muscles and therefore the overload on this muscle group would be compounded. This type of workout is specific to developing muscular endurance or hypertrophy rather than strength.

These types of workouts are not appropriate for novice exercisers or unconditioned fire fighters.

SAMPLE SUPERSET WORKOUT

This superset routine, which also happens to be a circuit training routine, is designed for the fire fighter with limited time. This routine can be performed three times per week and trains the entire body during every workout. This routine is not designed for maximum strength gains, rather it emphasizes both strength and endurance gains. The sets, repetitions, weights, days, and exercises may be modified to meet specific needs. Cardiovascular, abdominal, and flexibility exercises are also recommended for a total program.

Superset Workout Template

Group	Exercise	Weight	Repetitions	Sets
1	Leg Press	70% 1RM	10	3
1	Abdominal Crunches	Body weight	20	3
2	Seated Pulley Row	70% 1RM	10	3
2	Bench Press	70% 1RM	10	3
3	DB Row	70% 1RM	10	3
3	Pec Deck	70% 1RM	10	3
4	Single-Leg Leg Press	70% 1RM	10	3
4	Back Hyperextensions	Body weight	15	3
5	Chin-Ups	70% 1RM	10	3
5	DB Incline Bench	70% 1RM	10	3
6	V-Bar Pull Down	70% 1RM	10	3
6	Cable Crossovers	70% 1RM	10	3
7	Leg Extension	70% 1RM	10	3
7	Leg Curl	70% 1RM	10	3
8	EZ-Curl-Bar Curls	70% 1RM	10	3
8	Standing Tricep Extensions	70% 1RM	10	3
9	DB Seated Curls	70% 1RM	10	3
9	DB Kickbacks	70% 1RM	10	3

SAMPLE COMPOUND SET WORKOUT

Following is a compound set workout designed for the well-conditioned fire fighter who desires an intense workout. This routine can be performed two to three times per week and trains the entire body during every session. This workout is a circuit training routine and can be split by changing exercise order. Similarly, the workout can be split by grouping exercises and changing rest periods between exercises. This routine is not designed for maximum strength gains, rather it is designed to increase muscular hypertrophy and endurance. The sets, repetitions, weights, days, and exercises can be changed to meet specific needs. Cardiovascular, abdominal, and flexibility exercises are also recommended for a total program.

Compound Set Workout Template

Group	Exercise	Weight	Repetitions	Sets
1	Leg Press	70% 1RM	10	3
1	DB Single Squat	20 lbs.	10	3
2	Seated Pulley Row	70% 1RM	10	3
2	DB Row	70%1RM	10	3
3	Bench Press	70% 1RM	10	3
3	Pec Deck	70% 1RM	10	3
4	Single-Leg Press	70% 1RM	10	3
4	Leg Extension	70% 1RM	10	3
5	Chin-Ups	70% 1RM	10	3
5	V-Bar Pull Down	70% 1RM	10	3
6	DB Incline Bench	70% 1RM	10	3
6	Cable Crossovers	70% 1RM	10	3
7	EZ-Curl-Bar Curls	70% 1RM	10	3
7	DB Seated Curls	70% 1RM	10	3
8	Standing Tricep Extensions	70% 1RM	10	3
8	DB Kickbacks	70% 1RM	10	3

CIRCUIT TRAINING

Circuit training is a method of resistance training designed to increase muscular strength, muscular endurance, and cardiovascular endurance simultaneously. It contains numerous exercises that are performed one immediately after the other with little or no rest between exercises. The number of times the circuit is repeated depends on the goals and experience of the fire fighter. The entire body can be trained by varying the muscle group exercised. The weight and repetitions can be altered to emphasize muscular strength, muscular endurance, or cardiovascular endurance.

Circuit training can be performed on duty with the entire crew, completed in an hour or less, designed to simulate fire fighting tasks with limited equipment, and easily varied. Circuits can even be designed to include cardiovascular exercises to further improve cardiorespiratory fitness. Circuit training is an efficient and varied way of strength training.

Almost any type of workout (e.g., superset, compound set) can be designed into a circuit. In addition, all types of exercises (e.g., agility, speed, plyometrics, balance) can be incorporated into the circuit. The following are examples of circuit training programs.

SAMPLE CIRCUIT TRAINING WORKOUT #1

Circuit training workouts may be performed on duty by an entire crew. They are ideal for fire fighters more interested in total-body fitness than maximum strength gains. Initially, a circuit is performed one time. As each fire fighter improves, he or she repeats the workout, eventually working up to a maximum of three times. The sets, repetitions, weights, and exercises can be changed to meet specific needs. Cardiovascular, abdominal, and flexibility exercises are also recommended for a total program. Table 7.3 illustrates a sample circuit training workout.

Table 7.3 Sample Circuit Workout #1

Exercise	Date:								
	Wt	Wt	Wt	Wt	Wt	Wt	Wt	Wt	Wt
1. Treadmill at 60% max HR for 2 minutes									
2. Bench Press, 10 repetitions									
3. DB Rows, 10 repetitions									
4. Bike @ 70% max HR for 2 minutes									
5. DB Military Press, Standing, 10 repetitions									
6. Lat Pull-Down, Anterior, Wide Grip, 10 reps									
7. Treadmill at 70% max HR for 2 minutes									
8. Push Ups, 25 repetitions									
9. Posterior DB Flyes, 10 repetitions									
10. Bike at 70% max HR for 2 minutes									
11. Alternating DB Curls, 15 repetitions									
12. Standing Tricep Extensions, 15 repetitions									
13. Treadmill at 70% max HR for 2 minutes									

SAMPLE CIRCUIT TRAINING WORKOUT #2

This circuit workout also can be performed on duty by an entire crew. It is ideal for fire fighters who want constant action, are interested in total fitness more than maximum strength, have limited time, and can handle high-intensity workouts. Initially, this circuit can be performed one time. As each fire fighter improves, he or she repeats each of the mini circuits, eventually working up to a maximum of three times. The sets, repetitions, weights, and exercises can be changed to meet specific needs. Cardiovascular, abdominal, and flexibility exercises are also recommended for a total program. This is a very advanced workout and should be implemented gradually.

Table 7.4 Sample Circuit Workout #2

Exercise	Date:									
1 Treadmill 5 minutes at 70% max HR										
		Weight	Reps	Weight	Reps	Weight	Reps	Weight	Reps	Weight	Reps
2 One-Leg DB Squats			10		10		10		10		10
2 Flat DB Bench			10		10		10		10		10
2 DB Bent-Over Rows			10		10		10		10		10

* repeat above mini circuit 3 times

3 Treadmill 5 minutes at 80% max HR										
		Weight	Reps	Weight	Reps	Weight	Reps	Weight	Reps	Weight	Reps
4 Leg Extension			10		10		10		10		10
4 Leg Curl			10		10		10		10		10
4 Incline DB Bench (35° of incline)			10		10		10		10		10
4 V-Bar Pull-Downs			10		10		10		10		10

* repeat above mini circuit 3 times

5 Treadmill 5 minutes at 75% max HR										
		Weight	Reps	Weight	Reps	Weight	Reps	Weight	Reps	Weight	Reps
6 Back DB Flyes (Posterior Delts)			10		10		10		10		10
6 Standing DB Military Press			10		10		10		10		10
6 DB Curls			10		10		10		10		10
6 Standing Tricep Extensions			10		10		10		10		10

* repeat above mini circuit 3 times

HELPFUL CIRCUIT TRAINING HINTS

1. Warm up properly with a couple of minutes on the bike and some light stretches.
2. Move immediately from the treadmill to the weights.
3. Choose a weight and perform 12 to 15 repetitions the first set.
4. Move immediately from each exercise to the next.
5. Use proper form on every repetition of every lift, reducing weight if necessary.

VARYING THE WORKOUTS

Although any well-designed resistance training program improves fitness and performance, the returns will eventually diminish. Eventually, physical and psychological adaptations occur less frequently, performance improvements diminish, and there is an increased risk of overtraining. At that time, exercises chosen, intensity, and volume must be modified. Periodization is a well-documented approach to building this variation into planned cycles (Table 7.5).

Table 7.5 Traditional Periodization Model for Athletes

Period	Preparation			Competition
Phase	Hypertrophy/Endurance	Basic Strength	Strength/Power	Peaking
Intensity	Low to moderate	High	High	Very high
Volume	High to moderate	Moderate	Low	Very Low
	3–6 sets	3–5 sets	3–5 sets	1–3 sets
	10–20 repetitions	4–6 repetitions	2–5 repetitions	1–3 repetitions

Adapted, by permission, from D. Wathen, T.R. Baechle, and R.W. Earle, 2000, "Training variation: periodization" in *Essentials of Strength Training and Conditioning*, 2nd ed., NSCA, edited by T.R. Baechle & R.W. Earle (Champaign, IL: Human Kinetics), 519.

The traditional periodization model is based upon improving athletic performance. This model is based upon a linear approach to having an athlete peak on a certain competition day and is very successful for training competitive athletes but less applicable to training fire fighters, for whom every shift may be a form of competition (i.e., working fire, major incident) (Garhammer, 1979; Stone & O'Bryant, 1987; Stone et al., 1981; Stone et al., 1982).

This model consists of macrocycles that typically last one full year. Each macrocycle is further broken into several mesocycles, each lasting several weeks to months. Athletic seasons are commonly divided into mesocycles corresponding to preseason, in-season, postseason, and off-season. Within each mesocycle are microcycles that typically last one to four weeks. This short cycle focuses on daily and weekly training variations. This linear model of training, while very effective, can become complicated and has limited application in the fire service outside the training academy environment.

Because of a fire fighter's work schedule, job demands, and need for simplicity, another non-linear periodization model is more appropriate. In this non-linear model, the focus is on daily fluctuations in load and volume for the core exercises. Heavy, light, and medium intensity days are incorporated within a weekly workout in the example shown in Table 7.6. This can be accomplished with or without changing training volume, depending on the number of repetitions performed. A common mistake is to lower the weight, increase the number of repetitions, and still perform to failure. This actually increases the intensity and may lead to diminished returns, decreased performance, overtraining, and possibly injury (Baker et al., 1994; Fleck & Kraemer, 1997; Poliquin, 1988).

Table 7.6 Nonlinear Periodization Model

Day	Monday	Wednesday	Friday
Intensity	Heavy	Light*	Medium**
Weight	85 to 95% 1RM	60 to 70% 1RM	70 to 80% 1RM
Repetitions	1 to 3	10	4 to 6

* very important that the 10th repetition is fairly easy   ** very important that the 10th repetition is not at failure

Another effective method is changing the exercises. When the body adapts to a particular exercise through developing neural patterns, the actual overload on the involved muscles can decrease. This requires change in exercises to challenge the neuromuscular systems to adapt. Change the exercises performed every three to six weeks. For example, replace the barbell bench press with the dumbbell bench press.

Another periodization method changes the exercises for the same workout performed on different days within the same week. For example, on Monday clients perform the barbell bench press and dumbbell incline bench press for the chest, but on Thursday clients perform the barbell incline bench press and the cable crossover. All of these exercises recruit the chest muscles but in slightly different motor patterns.

SAMPLE SPLIT-ROUTINE WORKOUT
FOUR-DAY SPLIT ROUTINE

Tuesday

Exercise	Weight	Repetitions	Sets
Squats	80% 1RM	8-10	5
Leg Extension	80% 1RM	8-10	3
Leg Curl	80% 1RM	8-10	3
Calf Raises	80% 1RM	8-10	5

Friday

Exercise	Weight	Repetitions	Sets
Leg Press	80% 1RM	8-10	5
Single-Leg DB Lunge	80% 1RM	8-10	3
Stiff Legged Deadlift	80% 1RM	8-10	3
Calf Raises	80% 1RM	8-10	3

Monday

Exercise	Weight	Repetitions	Sets
Flat Bench Barbell	80% 1RM	8-10	3
Seated Row	80% 1RM	8-10	3
Incline Bench	80% 1RM	8-10	3
V-Bar Pull-Downs	80% 1RM	8-10	3
DB Lateral Raises	80% 1RM	8-10	3
EZ-curl-bar curls	80% 1RM	8-10	3
Standing Tricep Extensions	80% 1RM	8-10	3
Abdominal Crunches	Bodyweight	25	3

Thursday

Exercise	Weight	Repetitions	Sets
DB Incline Bench	80% 1RM	8-10	3
DB Row	80% 1RM	8-10	3
Cable Crossover	80% 1RM	8-10	3
Wide Grip Pull-Downs	80% 1RM	8-10	3
Upright Row	80% 1RM	8-10	3
Alternating DB Curls	80% 1RM	8-10	3
Supine Tricep Extensions	80% 1RM	8-10	3
Abdominal Crunches	Bodyweight	25	3

Changing the exercises performed on a regular basis has another benefit for fire fighters. Since it is almost impossible to replicate fire fighting movements with weight exercises, it is important to strengthen all joints of the body in numerous planes. This is accomplished by using variations of exercises that all stimulate the same muscle group. An excellent resource for alternative exercises is Bill Pearl's *Keys to the Inner Universe* (Pearl, 1992).

REFERENCES

Baechle, T.R. & Earle, R. (2000). *Essentials of Strength Training and Conditioning*, 2nd Ed. Champaign, Ill.: Human Kinetics.

Baechle, T.R. & Groves, B.R. (1998) *Weight Training: Steps to Success*, 2nd Ed. Champaign, Ill.: Human Kinetics.

Baker, D. et al. (1994). Periodization: The effect on strength of manipulating volume and intensity. *Journal of Strength and Conditioning Research*, 8, 235–242.

Fleck, S.J. & Kraemer, W.J. (1997). *Designing Resistance Training Programs*, 2nd Ed. Champaign, Ill. Human Kinetics.

Garhammer, J. (1987). Periodization of strength training for athletes. *Track Techniques*, 73, 2398–2399.

Gettman, L.R. & Pollock, M.J. (1981). Circuit weight training: A critical review of its physiological benefits. *Physician and Sportsmedicine*, 9, 44–60.

Jones, A. (1971) *Nautilus Training Principles* (Bulletin No. 2), Deland, Fla.: Nautilus.

Kraemer, W.J. et al. (1995). Varied multiple set resistance training programs produce greater gain than single set programs. *Medicine and Science in Sports and Exercise*, 27, S195.

Kramer, J.B. et al. (1997). Effects of single vs. multiple sets of weight training: Impact on volume, intensity, and variation. *Journal of Strength and Conditioning Research*, 11, 3, 143–147.

Luthi, J.M. et al. (1986). Structural changes in skeletal muscle tissue with heavy resistance exercise. *International Journal of Sports Medicine*, 7, 123–127.

Pearl, B. (1992). *Keys to the Inner Universe*. Phoenix, Ore.: Bill Pearl Enterprises.

Pocock et al. (1989). Muscle strength, physical fitness, and weight but not age to predict femoral neck bone mass, *Journal of Bone Mineral Research*, 4, 3, 441–448.

Poliquin, C. (1998). Five steps to increasing the effectiveness of your strength training program. *National Strength and Conditioning Association Journal*, 10, 3, 34–39.

Stone, M.H. &. O'Bryant, H.S. (1987) *Weight Training: A Scientific Approach*. Edina, Minn.: Burgess International.

Stone, M.H. et al. (1982). A theoretical model for strength training. *National Strength and Conditioning Association Journal*, 4, 4, 36–40.

Stone, M.H. et al. (1981). A hypothetical model for strength training. *Journal of Sports Medicine and Physical Fitness*, 21, 336, 342–351.

Westcott, W.L. (1986). Four key factors in building a strength program. *Scholastic Coach*, 55, 104–105.

EXERCISE
EQUIPMENT

When selecting the type of fitness equipment for a given facility, several factors should be considered: space, pattern of use, safety, and transferability of training to job task.

EQUIPMENT FOR CARDIOVASCULAR CONDITIONING

The single most widely used piece of equipment in the fitness industry is the treadmill. Typically requiring an approximate area of 24 square feet, this piece of equipment is often a keystone of the fitness facility. When advising your department on treadmill selection, be sure to consider the type and amount of use it will have to withstand. Commercial grade treadmills are manufactured for heavy use with minimal maintenance. Most commercial treadmill makers offer some type of flexible deck, and there is some variety in the belts and motors offered. Research your options before simply accepting the lowest bid.

In rooms where space is at an absolute premium, stair steppers allow for minimal to maximal intensities of exercise, but require roughly half the space of a treadmill.

Steppers are not as likely to be used as treadmills, however, as the movement is less familiar. Some users may complain of knee pain while using a stepper, while others find that it produces lower impact exercise than walking or running. The StairMaster StepMill 7000 PT that is used in the CPAT operates like a vertical treadmill and simulates actual stair climbing very well. Other steppers allow the user to adjust the step height but have less transferability to actual stair climbing.

Another popular piece of cardiovascular equipment is the elliptical trainer, or cross trainer. Several equipment companies offer elliptical trainers with slight variations in design. An advantage of

CHAPTER

these trainers is that they produce a variety of workouts with little or no impact on the ankles, knees, or lower back. Several of the models offer combination leg and arm workouts while others include incline capabilities. Elliptical trainers require a similar amount of space as a treadmill and can be less expensive. Where possible, offer one of these three weightbearing options for cardiovascular exercise, because they require greater energy expenditure than non-weightbearing equipment (such as stationary cycles or rowing machines).

EQUIPMENT FOR STRENGTH TRAINING

Space is also an important consideration in the selection of strength equipment. The multi-station "gym" is the most compact way to exercise all the major muscle groups. A single piece of equipment can provide from two to six workout stations. The limitation of multi-station gyms is that the number of users cannot exceed the number of weight stacks it incorporates, so be sure it is designed to handle the expected use. Units that are designed for "home" gyms usually do not withstand the wear and tear of fire station use and often do not provide enough resistance. While many of these multi-station units may be similar in appearance, the workmanship, biomechanics, bearings, pulleys, levers, and cable systems can vary significantly. Several equipment manufacturers offer single station units with numerous adjustable pulleys that can be utilized for many exercises.

A variety of single-station machines can accommodate the greatest number of people. This tends to be the most expensive option, requiring considerable space if there are units for all major muscle groups. Single station machines work for departments that opt to build central exercise facilities. Again, be sure to purchase equipment that is designed for heavy use.

Free weights can be placed in a relatively small space, and can easily accommodate multiple users. An Olympic rack, a multi-angle bench, and a set of dumbbells can be used simultaneously by several users. In a multi-company fire station, free weights are probably the best option for strength training because they are compact and economical.

Strength machines are the safest choice, because the range of motion is limited mechanically and the weights are in fixed positions. Conversely, free weights must be controlled by muscular work through the entire range of motion and may cause injuries if dropped. However, the "freedom of movement" inherent in free weight exercise can produce positive effects. Muscle stabilizers and synergists are recruited during free weight use, so proprioception can be improved. Free weight exercises may also be designed to resemble job tasks.

In summary, no single option for equipping an exercise room exists. Although budget and space are frequently the limiting factors, there are several other important factors, including the number of simultaneous users, the nature of the work, the durability of the equipment, and the level of instruction and supervision the facility can provide. For more information regarding names and addresses of equipment manufacturers contact:

Fitness Management Products & Services Source Guide
PO Box 10295
Riverton, NJ 08076-8795
http://www.fitnessworld.com

For more information regarding facility design and space guidelines refer to *ASCM's Health/Fitness Facility Standards and Guidelines*, Second Edition (American College of Sports Medicine, 1997).

WARRANTY OF EQUIPMENT

Regardless of the pieces chosen for the fire station fitness equipment complement, it is highly advisable to include a full commercial warranty. A full commercial warranty is distinguished from other types of manufacturer warranties by the setting in which it is to be used, and the amount of use expected.

A "home" or "retail" warranty is typically provided on equipment used by one or two individuals in a residential setting. This type of warranty typically does not cover damage to equipment, nor does the manufacturer's liability insurance cover injury to a user when it is placed in a fire station setting. The type of equipment covered by a home warranty is not intended to stand up to the high demands of station use.

Equipment dealers may submit bids for equipment covered by a "light commercial" warranty. Light commercial equipment is designed for a setting in which it is used no more than four hours per day. Commercial equipment, on the other hand, is constructed to stand up to more than four hours of continual use per day such as the equipment in health clubs or gyms. Commercial equipment manufacturers typically repair or replace equipment that malfunctions during the term of the warranty. All reputable fitness equipment manufacturers hold product liability insurance in the event a user is injured due to equipment failure or malfunction.

Fire department responsibilities are not limited to equipment selection. Departments must also allow adequate space for both the equipment and the number of people likely to work out at one time. Weight stacks, moving cables, lever arms, bars, and electrical cords all represent potential for injury unless plenty of passing room is provided. There should be at least three feet of space between each piece of equipment.

Another responsibility of the department, and very likely the PFT, is to inspect the equipment at regular intervals. Frayed cables or electrical cords, torn upholstery, and malfunctioning joints or bearings all represent dangers to the user. When equipment irregularities or malfunctions are discovered, the equipment should be removed from service immediately until it is repaired by a qualified technician.

PFTs must ensure that all equipment is kept clean. Daily cleaning of upholstery and mats with an antibacterial cleaner for non-porous materials minimizes the risk of bacterial or fungal skin infections. A simple cleaning solution of water, soap, and 10% household bleach may also be used. All other equipment, such as aerobic exercise machines, weight racks, and equipment without upholstery, should be wiped down thoroughly at least once a week.

REFERENCE

American College of Sports Medicine. (1997). *ACSM's Health/Fitness Facility Standards and Guidelines*, 2nd ed. Champaign, Ill.: Human Kinetics.

FLEXIBILITY TRAINING

Despite the fact that flexibility exercise is perhaps the easiest fitness component to modify, it is the most frequently overlooked. PFTs should communicate to clients the importance of budgeting time for flexibility training. A flexibility training program is a planned, deliberate, regular program of specific stretching exercises that progressively increases the usable and functional range of motion of a joint or set of joints over a period of time. Flexibility is not only the ability of a joint to move freely through a full range of motion, but is also the ability to contract and recover without injury. Flexibility differs from person to person and from joint to joint on the same person. Flexibility encompasses all components of the musculoskeletal system as well as specific neuromuscular pathways of the body. The primary benefit of participating in a flexibility training program is *reduction in the risk of injury.*

Stretching exercises are typically performed during the warm-up and/or cool-down components of workouts or athletic events. Stretching during warm-up and cool-down serves different purposes and PFTs must understand the difference. Warm-up is a group of exercises or activities performed immediately before an activity, providing mind and body with a period of adjustment from rest to exercise. In general, stretches performed during warm-up should be light to moderate with the goal of lengthening muscle fibers and preparing them for the activity to follow. Cool-down is a group of exercises or movements performed immediately after an activity that provides a period of adjustment from exercise to rest. In general, stretches performed during this time should be deeper and longer to promote long-term increases in flexibility.

CHAPTER

WARM-UP

An effective warm-up consists of the following two phases.

Phase 1: General Warm-Up. This phase consists of 5 to 10 minutes of activity such as stationary cycling, fast walking, jogging, or light calisthenics. The intensity should be enough to increase the body core temperature and cause light sweating, but not cause fatigue.

Phase 2: Specific Warm-Up or Pre-Stretch. The specific warm-up phase involves 5 to 10 minutes of movements that either mimic or are similar to actual performance of the activity to follow. Ideally, this phase includes light sport-specific stretches. The stretching techniques that are most effective during this pre-stretch phase are held less than 10 seconds or are controlled dynamic stretches throughout a range of motion. These techniques are discussed in detail later in this section. This phase is often called the pre-stretch and is somewhat controversial. Many experts claim that the pre-stretch prevents injury. However, some studies show that many athletes and fitness enthusiasts who do not regularly stretch prior to exercise or activity have the same rate or fewer injuries compared to those who perform a pre-stretch prior to exercise or activity. The most important undisputed benefit of the pre-stretch is that *it feels good*, and clients report that they feel more physically and mentally prepared to exercise. The biggest misconception is that stretching *is* the warm-up. The pre-stretch can be an optional part of the warm-up and should never replace the general warm-up.

COOL-DOWN

The cool-down provides many benefits: it facilitates muscular relaxation, promotes the removal of metabolic waste products, reduces muscle soreness, and allows the cardiovascular system to adjust to lowered demand. The cool-down is a group of exercises or movements performed immediately after an activity that provides the mind and body with a period of adjustment from exercise to rest. The cool-down is the optimal time to improve long-term flexibility due to the increased muscle temperature created during the activity. Stretching exercises should be performed within 5 to 10 minutes after the activity to take advantage of increased muscle temperature. Effective techniques include stretches held for 20 seconds or more, proprioceptive neuromuscular facilitation (PNF), and other various techniques that are low force, long duration. These techniques are discussed in detail later in this chapter.

BENEFITS

The benefits of participating in a flexibility training program are numerous, including:

- Increased physical efficiency and performance (Taylor et al., 1990)
- Increased neuromuscular coordination (Beaulieu, 1980)
- Increased enjoyment and sense of well-being (Alter, 1988)
- Decreased risk of incidence and severity of injury (Safran et al., 1988)

- Decreased risk of lower back pain (Bach, et al., 1985: Farfan, 1973)
- Decreased muscle soreness (de Vries, 1961)
- Decreased onset of muscle soreness (de Vries & Adams, 1972)
- Decreased stress and tension (de Vries et al., 1981)

PHYSIOLOGICAL FACTORS LIMITING FLEXIBILITY

There are numerous physiological factors that influence flexibility, including joint structure and muscle reflexes. When a muscle is relaxed and reflex mechanics are minimally involved, the relative contributions to flexibility potential are as follows: joint capsule, including ligaments (47%), muscles and fascia sheaths (41%), tendons (10%), and skin (2%) (Johns & Wright, 1962). Thus, problems with joints and connective tissue may limit clients' flexibility potential.

JOINT STRUCTURE

Ultimately, the range of motion of a joint is restricted by its structure. There are three types of joints, categorized according to the amount of movement they allow.

- *Synarthroses* – immoveable joints, such as cranial sutures
- *Amphiarthroses* – slightly movable joints, such as sacroiliac
- *Diarthroses* – freely movable joints, such as the elbows

MUSCLE SENSORY REFLEXES

There are specialized sensory receptors in muscles, joints, and ligaments that are sensitive to stretch, tension, and pressure. These sensors rapidly relay information concerning limb movement to the central nervous system. All body movements are continually monitored by these neuromuscular receptors.

Reflexes are automatic responses designed to protect the body, such as the patellar reflex (knee jerk) and the automatic reflex to pull away from something hot. There are three specific muscular reflexes that are related to stretching: stretch reflex, inverse stretch reflex, and reciprocal inhibition.

The stretch reflex prevents a muscle from stretching too far and/or too fast, thereby protecting the joint and muscle from injury. Muscle spindles are located in the muscle belly (see page 309 of the *ACE Personal Trainer Manual* for an illustration of muscle spindles). Their function is to sense changes in muscle length and speed of changes as summarized in Table 9.1. When the spindle is stimulated, it causes the muscle to contract to prevent over-stretching. During static stretching, the spindle is stretched, causing the muscle to contract. Over time, the reflex dissipates, allowing the muscle to elongate. During a sudden (ballistic) stretch, a very forceful contraction of the stretched muscle occurs in a fraction of a second.

The inverse stretch reflex is controlled by the Golgi tendon organs (GTOs), which are located in the muscle tendons (see page 309 of the *ACE Personal Trainer Manual* for an illustration of GTOs). GTOs monitor the amount of strain or tension in the muscle and tendon during muscle contraction and stretching as summarized in Table 9.1. When the GTOs fire, they cause the muscle to relax. It is theorized that a muscle is neurologically relaxed, and therefore more easily stretched, following a maximal isometric contraction. When a muscle stretch is held, the pull on the tendons should stimulate the GTOs, causing the muscle to relax and lengthen, and reducing the chances of muscle tearing.

Table 9.1 A Summary of Muscle Spindles and Golgi Tendon Organs

	Location	Responds to…	Function	Protects…
Muscle Spindles	Muscle belly	Speed and length of stretch	Causes muscle to contract	Muscles from injury
Golgi Tendon Organs (GTOs)	Muscle-tendon junction	Tension in the muscle	Causes muscle to relax	Muscles and tendons from injury

Reciprocal inhibition is the third reflex. It is a reflex loop started by muscle spindle cells that causes one muscle to relax when an opposing muscle contracts. For example, when the quads contract, the hamstrings are reciprocally inhibited, thereby allowing the knee to straighten and the hamstrings to relax. This is an easy technique to incorporate into stretching exercises by simply contracting the antagonist muscle to the targeted muscle to be stretched. The target muscle will automatically relax and lengthen.

FACTORS THAT INFLUENCE FLEXIBILITY POTENTIAL

❑ Past and Current Injuries
   Injuries can decrease joint range of motion temporarily, and sometimes permanently. Lack of activity, usually associated with injury, also causes loss of flexibility.

❑ Lifestyle and Current Activity Level
   A sedentary lifestyle usually results in loss of flexibility. Regular participation in physical activity involving full range of motion generally enhances flexibility (Beaulieu, 1980).

❑ Body Composition, Body Type
   Range of motion is not affected by arm or leg length, arm span, height, or weight. An obese person may be very flexible, but the sit-and-reach score may be low due to adipose tissue in the abdominal area, which mechanically inhibits movement (Alter, 1988).

❑ Age
   The aging process involves a loss in elasticity of connective tissues, including tissues surrounding muscles. Regular exercise and participation in activity can minimize age-related muscle shortening and loss of flexibility (Chapman et al., 1972).

❑ Gender
At any age, females tend to be more flexible than males. This is probably due to anatomical variations in joint structures (Holland, 1968).

❑ Pregnancy
During pregnancy, the hormone relaxin causes the pelvic joints and tendons to relax and therefore increase range of motion for the birth process. Relaxin affects all joints in the pregnant woman and is usually present for six weeks or more postpartum (Bird et al., 1981).

❑ Muscle Temperature
Increase in body temperature due to participation in physical activity increases range of motion. Lowering body temperature results in decreased flexibility (Sapega et al., 1981).

❑ Ability to Relax
Reduction in internal tension facilitates elongation of connective tissue (Alter, 1988).

❑ Resistance Training
Resistance exercises using full range of motion may improve flexibility (Massey & Chaudet, 1956).

STRETCHING TECHNIQUES

The goal of all stretching is to optimize joint mobility while maintaining joint stability. There are many stretching techniques that can be used in flexibility training programs. There are numerous books and articles by experts who claim that their technique is the most effective way to increase flexibility. Improvements in flexibility can be produced by all techniques of stretching if they are performed on a regular basis. The basic techniques are static, dynamic (ballistic and controlled dynamic), and PNF stretching. Each stretching technique uses passive stretching (relaxing), active stretching (contracting), or a combination of both. Passive and active stretching principles are described first, followed by the use of these principles in static, dynamic, and PNF techniques.

PASSIVE (RELAX)

In passive stretching, the individual's muscles do not generate the stretching force. Instead, the stretching motion is performed by an outside agent, such as a partner or piece of equipment such as a strap, rope, ballet bar, or the floor. The stretch can be within or beyond the normal functional range of motion as when attempting to increase the permanent range of motion.

ACTIVE (CONTRACT)

In active stretching, the individual uses his or her own muscle contraction to perform the stretch without aid. The muscles produce the movement without application of additional external resistance. Voluntary muscle contractions can also be made against an applied resistance, such as a partner or machine.

COMBINATION OF PASSIVE AND ACTIVE

In passive-active stretching, the stretch begins with muscles relaxed and a partner or piece of equipment initiating the range of motion. Then, that range of motion is held only by the muscle contraction of the individual.

In active-passive stretching, the stretch begins with the individual contracting either the target muscle or the antagonist muscle, and a partner or piece of equipment is used to increase the range of motion as the muscles relax. This is the most popular method used in PNF.

STATIC

Static stretching is the safest and most common method of stretching. It involves slow and controlled muscle elongation held at an "end point." The stretch is held for a period of time ranging from 10 to 60 seconds or more. Static stretching is low intensity, long duration. The advantages are that it is easy to perform, increases range of motion, and enhances relaxation. The disadvantage is that is does not usually produce an increase in dynamic range of motion. Static stretching can be active, passive, or a combination of both.

DYNAMIC

Dynamic stretching is movement through a range of motion. The movement can be ballistic or controlled. Dynamic stretching can be active, passive, or a combination of both.

BALLISTIC

Ballistic stretching involves dynamic movements of high force and short duration. Ballistic stretches may appear to be rapid bouncing or bobbing. This type of stretching can be appropriate and functional for specific sports, such as martial arts and punt kicks, and specific job-related skills. However, it is commonly considered unsafe and is likely to cause injury if not performed properly. Clients should prepare by thoroughly warming up and executing several slow pre-stretches.

Ballistic stretching should only be performed when training for a specific sport or skill that uses similar ballistic action. When performing ballistic stretching, adhere to the principle of Specific Adaptation to Imposed Demands (SAID). The SAID principle states that one should stretch at the same velocity, through the exact range of motion, and at the precise joint angles as when performing the sport or skill. Ballistic stretching should not be used for cool-down.

CONTROLLED DYNAMIC

Controlled dynamic stretching is a slow and controlled movement through a range of motion, not holding at an end point. It is often used by athletes to increase sport-specific flexibility. It is also used in group exercise classes during the specific warm-up segment. It gives a feeling of readiness, while keeping the energy high and heart rate up. It is low-force and short-duration.

The advantages are that it involves a functional range of motion and feels good prior to exercise. The disadvantage is that it is difficult to increase long-term flexibility with this type of stretching, as it is typically performed only during the warm-up.

PROPRIOCEPTIVE NEUROMUSCULAR FACILITATION

Proprioceptive neuromuscular facilitation (PNF) is a popular stretching technique that is usually done with a partner, trainer, or therapist. Many PNF stretches can be done by an individual using a strap or towel for assistance. PNF is an advanced technique and utilizes contract/relax (active/passive) stretches. Communication between partners is vital. The advantage is that PNF is very effective in increasing range of motion. However, this method requires thorough knowledge of proper techniques and effective trainer/client communication.

PNF Techniques

A wide variety of techniques can be used in PNF stretching. Nine different PNF techniques are discussed in Michael J. Alter's *Science of Flexibility* (2000). The techniques include various isotonic and isometric contractions in different combinations. Additionally, contractions of agonist and antagonist muscles may be included.

The two most common PNF techniques are contract-relax and contract-relax-agonist contract. Both are simple and can be used individually or with a skilled partner. Partners must communicate effectively and understand the protocol to be used.

PNF/Contract-Relax

- Stretch the target muscle to the end point.

- Using the partner or strap for resistance, isometrically contract the stretched muscle for four to eight seconds.

- Relax the contracted target muscle and gently move it to a new end point.

- Repeat two to three times, starting at the new end point.

❑ **Example of the PNF hamstrings stretch: Contract-Relax**

Lying prone on the floor, bend the left knee with the left foot flat on the floor and the right leg straight on the floor. Using a partner, or a strap or towel around the foot or leg, relax the quadriceps and pull the straight right leg toward the head and hold for a few moments. Stretch the hamstrings to the end point. Using the partner or strap for resistance, isometrically contract the hamstring muscles for four to eight seconds. Relax the hamstring muscles and gently move to a new end point. Repeat two to three times, starting at the new end point.

PNF/Contract-Relax-Agonist Contract

- Stretch the target muscle to the end point.

- Using the partner or strap for resistance, isometrically contract the stretched muscle for 6 to 10 seconds.

- Relax the contracted target muscle and gently move it to a new end point

- Using the partner or strap for resistance, isometrically contract the agonist muscle (opposite the target muscle) for four to eight seconds.

- Release the agonist contraction and move the target muscle to a new end point.

- Repeat two to three times, starting at the new end point.

❑ **Example of PNF hamstrings stretch: Contract-Relax-Agonist Contract**

Lying prone on the floor, bend the left knee with the left foot flat on the floor and the right leg straight on the floor. Using a partner, or a strap or towel around the foot or leg, relax the quadriceps and pull the straight right leg toward the head and hold for a few moments. Stretch the hamstrings to the end point. Using the partner or strap for resistance, isometrically contract the hamstring muscles for four to eight seconds. Relax the hamstring muscles and gently move to a new end point. Using the partner or strap for resistance, isometrically contract the quadriceps for four to eight seconds. Release the quadriceps and move the hamstrings stretch to a new end point. Repeat two to three times, starting at the new end point.

FLEXIBILITY TESTING

The purpose of flexibility testing is to record a baseline, motivate the client to improve, and evaluate the score relative to norms for age and gender. Typically, flexibility tests are performed in a static stretch position after the client has performed a warm-up. However, the less common "cold" flexibility test shows the everyday functional flexibility level. If you decide to use both methods with your client, document whether the test was performed with or without a warm-up for consistent follow-up testing.

The *ACE Personal Trainer Manual* describes numerous flexibility tests including trunk flexibility, sit and reach, trunk extension, shoulder flexibility, hamstrings flexibility, and hip flexion. The Wellness-Fitness Initiative protocol for trunk flexion is the modified sit and reach. It is described on page 79.

FLEXIBILITY TRAINING PROGRAM DESIGN

A flexibility training program is a planned, focused, regular program of specific stretching exercises that progressively increases the functional range of motion of a joint or set of joints over a period of time. Program components are listed in Table 9.2 and described in greater detail below.

Table 9.2 Flexibility Training Program Components: "FITT"

F	Frequency – How often will stretching be performed? How many times per day and/or days per week will the client participate in flexibility training?
I	Intensity – What is the intensity of the stretch?
T	Time – What is the duration of the stretch? How many sets?
T	Type – What type of stretching will be performed?

Adapted from American College of Sports Medicine. (2000). *ACSM's Guidelines for Exercise Testing and Prescription,* 6/e. Philadelphia: Lippincott, Williams & Wilkins.

F – FREQUENCY

ACSM Guidelines recommend a minimum of three times per week for specific flexibility training of major muscle and/or tendon groups. Three to four sets of the same muscle are optimal. Use a variety of stretches that target the same muscle. Perform light stretches as often as possible throughout the day, especially when muscles feel tight or tense.

I – INTENSITY

There are many different ways to describe intensity for stretching. Stretch to "the end point" or "to a position of mild discomfort." PFTs can also advise, "Train don't strain," "Listen to your body," and "Know your comfort zone." In all cases, use common sense, and know the goals and health conditions of your client.

T – TIME

The length of time to hold a stretch position is a controversial topic. Teach clients to listen to their bodies. As a rule of thumb, beginners are able to hold a stretch comfortably for a shorter period of time than someone who stretches on a regular basis. There is no absolute rule on how long to hold a stretch. Research indicates that range of motion is increased when the stretch is held for 10–30 seconds (American Council on Exercise, 2003; Taylor et al., 1990; American College of Sports Medicine, 2000). Other research indicates that the stretch should be held for 60 seconds or more to achieve increased range of motion (Bates, 1971; Anderson, 1980).

T – TYPE

PFTs should use a variety of techniques including static, controlled dynamic, and PNF stretching techniques. Regardless of the technique used for flexibility training, always start with a general, active warm-up to ensure safety and effectiveness. Perform at least 8 to 10 minutes of cardiovascular activity such as stationary cycling, fast walking, jogging, or light calisthenics. Whenever possible, perform a flexibility training program after the complete workout. Know the muscles and the muscle origin, insertion, and action to isolate the target muscle most effectively.

EVALUATING STRETCHES

There are hundreds of books on stretching and thousands of different stretches. PFTs must know how to evaluate the safety and effectiveness of stretches that have been learned from well-meaning high school coaches, physical education teachers, and from articles and books. Clients may have to unlearn improper techniques and ineffective stretches.

GUIDELINES FOR EVALUATING SAFETY AND EFFECTIVENESS OF EACH STRETCH

Consider each of the following issues when evaluating stretches:

❑ Safety is always the top priority. Not all stretches are safe and effective for everyone. Is there a safer position to target the same muscle? Are the risks higher than the benefits?

❑ Every stretch should have a specific purpose. What is the purpose of the stretch?

❑ Stretching should not cause extreme or sharp pain. Is the movement within a relatively normal range of motion? Is there hyperextension or impingement of any joint? Are the head, neck, and spine in neutral positions? Is the knee in extreme flexion? (Extreme flexion may cause patellofemoral pain.) Is the stretch using forward trunk flexion? (Avoid unsupported forward flexion of the spine in a standing position, especially with a twisting motion.) Are you compromising any part of the body?

❑ Never stretch:

• Areas near a fracture

• Areas recently sprained or strained

• Joints or muscles that are infected or inflamed, or are arthritic

• With clients who have osteoporosis, unless a physician gives specific recommendations

THE ROLE OF THE PEER FITNESS TRAINER

PFTs may be responsible for training both individual clients and groups within their fire departments. Providing flexibility instruction to a group of recruits can be challenging. It is important to consider several factors prior to developing and leading a group flexibility training program.

INTRODUCTION TO GROUP FLEXIBILITY PROGRAMS

Before leading a group in a flexibility program, discuss the benefits participants gain through flexibility training. PFTs should use the "FITT" mnemonic to guide them through the introduction. The introduction can be done in a classroom setting with the recruits viewing pictures of the stretches and the PFT demonstrating each of the stretches using the Tell-Show-Do teaching technique. As the PFT demonstrates each stretch, the muscles stretched should be identified so all members of the group understand the proper technique and the appropriate target muscle. The class members should also learn proper form of the stretches by practicing them, not simply by hearing the instructor describe them.

LENGTH OF SESSION

If the stretching session has no time constraints, choose a variety of stretches that encompass all of the major muscle groups of the body. If the session is limited in time, carefully select stretches for the muscles used most frequently by group members.

TIMING OF THE SESSION

PFTs should emphasize that stretching during warm-up is different than stretching during cooldown. Also, conducting group stretches on a cold morning produces a different effect than group stretches on a warm afternoon.

SELECTION OF STRETCHES

Stretch selection depends on the size of the group, the time allotted to the physical training portion of the recruit program, and the physical requirements of the tasks that the recruits will be performing that day. Although the best stretches might be the PNF type, it is difficult to use these stretches in a group because time is limited and recruits may lack experience. Choose stretches for the group that can be performed by all members of the group and focus on those muscle groups most often used and/or injured during training. The stretches found in the CPAT Physical Preparation Guide are an excellent place to begin when developing group flexibility training programs.

CLASS ORGANIZATION

A large group is obviously harder to instruct than a small group or an individual. Position of the instructor, participants' view of the instructor, effective cueing, voice projection, and supervision of form and position all make group instruction more difficult. The least effective class formation for instruction and learning is a circle with the leader in the middle. Although this formation is motivating to groups and teams familiar with the movements, it is not conducive to learning new skills. The most effective formation is with the instructor in full view of the students. If facing the class, the instructor should mirror the students. For example, the instructor facing the class will cue right leg but will use the left leg. Acquiring this teaching skill requires practice.

INSTRUCTION TECHNIQUES

Instruction techniques include effective cueing, voice projection, supervision of proper form, position correction, and positive feedback. Cueing and voice projection go hand-in-hand. PFTs must not only cue the stretch correctly, but also speak so that all participants can hear. Imagine cueing an individual who is vision-impaired to help you create awareness of verbal directions that are most effective.

Supervision of form and correction of positioning is probably the most important aspect of leading a group class. Each participant should have adequate room around them to perform the stretches properly. Immediately correct improper form to ensure safety and prevent risk of injury. Avoid embarrassing or belittling participants. Instead, use the following strategy to correct the position of a participant. First look in the direction of the participant and make a verbal correction to the entire class. If that is not effective, try taking a step or two toward the participant and re-wording the correction. If necessary, discretely move to the participant and make verbal corrections in a low tone of voice. Corrective cues should always be followed by positive feedback. Positive feedback ensures successful and motivated participants.

EMPOWERMENT

It is important to encourage recruits to take ownership of their flexibility training programs. To promote this ideal, recruit fitness leaders can lead the stretching sessions after PFTs have taught proper form and correct execution. Recruit fitness leaders can be responsible for leading the stretches by calling out the exercise and counts for each stretch. PFTs must be cautious when using this form of leadership. Recruits may choose stretches that are unsafe for the group. PFTs are the fitness experts, and are responsible for choosing appropriate stretches for each group. A flexibility routine in provided in Appendix 3-1 of the *CPAT Manual*.

REFERENCES

Alter, M.J. (1996). *Science of Flexibility*. Champaign, Ill.: Human Kinetics.

Alter, M.J. (1988). *Science of Stretching*. Champaign, Ill.: Human Kinetics.

American College of Sports Medicine. (2000). *ACSM's Guidelines for Exercise Testing and Prescription*, 6/e. Philadelphia: Lippincott, Williams & Wilkins.

American Council on Exercise. (2003). *ACE Personal Trainer Manual*, 3rd edition. San Diego: American Council on Exercise.

Anderson, B. (1980). *Stretching*. Bolinas, Cal.: Shelter.

Bach, B.K. et al. (1985). A comparison of muscular tightness in runners and non-runners and the relation of muscular tightness to low back pain in runners. *Journal of Orthopedic Sports Physical Therapy*, 6, 315–323.

Bates, R.A. (1971). *Flexibility training: The optimal time period to spend in a position of maximal stretch.* Unpublished master's thesis, University of Alberta, Edmonton.

Beaulieu, J.E. (1981). Developing a stretching program. *The Physician and Sportsmedicine*, 9, 11, 59–69.

Beaulieu, J.E. (1980). *Stretching for All Sports*. Pasadena, Cal.: Athletic Press.

Bird, H. A. et al. (1981). Changes in joint laxity occurring during pregnancy, *Annals of the Rheumatic Diseases*, 40, 209–212.

Chapman, E.A. et al. (1972). Joint stiffness: Effects of exercise of young and old men. *Journal of Gerontology*, 27, 2, 218–221.

de Vries, H.A., Wiswell, R.A., Bulbulion, R., & Moritani, T. (1981). Tranquilizer effect of exercise. *American Journal of Physical Medicine*, 60, 57–66.

de Vries, H.A. (1961). Electromyographic observation of the effect of static stretching upon muscular distress. *Research Quarterly*, 32, 4, 468–479.

de Vries, H.A. & Adams, G.M. (1972). EMG comparison of single doses of exercise and meprobamate as to effects on muscular relaxation. *American Journal of Physical Medicine*, 51, 3, 130–141.

Farfan, H.F. (1973). *Mechanical Disorders of the Low Back*. Philadelphia: Lea & Febiger.

Garrett, W. et al. (1989). Basic science perspectives. In J.W. Frymoyer and S.L. Gordon (Eds.), *New Perspectives in Low Back Pain* (pp. 335–372). Park Ridge, Ill.: Amercian Academy of Orthropaedic Surgeons.

Holland, G.J. (1968). The physiology of flexibility: A review of the literature. *Kinesiology Review*, 49–62.

Johns, R.J., & Wright, V. (1962). Relative importance of various tissues in joint stiffness. *Journal of Applied Physiology*, 17, 824–828.

Massey, B.A., & Chaudet, N.L. (1956). Effects of systematic, heavy, resistance exercise on range of movement in young adults. *Research Quarterly*, 27, 41–51.

Safran, M.R. et al. (1988). The role of warmup in muscular injury prevention. *The American Journal of Sports Medicine*, 16,123–129.

Sapega, A.A. et al. (1981). Biophysical factors in range-of-motion exercises. *The Physician and Sportsmedicine*, 9, 57–65.

Taylor, D. et al. (1990). Viscoelastic properties of muscle and tendon units – the biomechanical effects of stretching. *American Journal of Sports Medicine*, 18, 300–309.

GENERAL FITNESS PROGRAMMING

Successful fitness programming allows for individual needs and goals of fire fighters, as well as department resources. This chapter discusses key concepts of fitness programming and the unique needs of the specific categories of clients. It is especially important for PFTs to keep current in the fitness field to make the best program decisions.

GENERAL PROGRAMMING STEPS

When developing fitness programs for fire fighters, it is important to have an approach to programming that can be used in all circumstances. A standard approach will allow PFTs to develop programs for everyone from the fire fighter candidate preparing for the CPAT to the veteran fire fighter approaching retirement. The steps are summarized as follows.

Developing Fitness Programs for Fire Fighters

Step 1. Health Screening

Step 2. Determine the Fire Fighter's Goals and Preferences

Step 3. Determine Current Fitness Level

Step 4. Develop the Exercise Plan

Step 5. Implement the Plan

Step 6. Progress and Re-evaluate

HEALTH SCREENING

Health screening includes filling out a health history questionnaire (HHQ) to determine whether the fire fighter will need a medical clearance prior to any programming. If the fire department participates in the WFI, the fire fighter's yearly physical is sufficient medical clearance. The HHQ will also alert the PFT of any previous injury, which may affect exercise or fitness test selection.

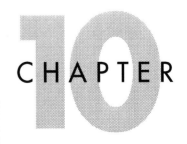

CHAPTER **10**

GOALS AND PREFERENCES

When developing a program, it is important to address the fire fighter's goals, the fire department's goals, as well as the job demands of fire fighting. In addition, perform the fire fighter's preferred modes of exercise as much as possible. For example, if a fire fighter reports that he or she hates running, the PFT should choose another cardiovascular activity to make the program complete.

CURRENT FITNESS LEVEL

In order to set goals for an exercise program, a PFT must first know the fire fighter's baseline fitness level. The WFI provides protocols for measurement of all aspects of fire fighter fitness. In the absence of equipment to utilize these protocols, a PFT must become familiar with alternate tests that measure fire fighters' baseline fitness levels.

THE EXERCISE PLAN

The exercise plan should be a complete program that addresses cardiovascular exercise, muscular strength, muscular endurance, and flexibility. How much or how little of each aspect is dependant on the overall goal of the program and the fire fighters' current strengths and weaknesses, which were determined in the baseline testing.

IMPLEMENT THE PLAN

The plan is a guideline and should be followed as closely as possible. However, the PFT should be prepared to adapt the program due to unforeseen circumstances such as injuries, illnesses, and fire fighter fatigue unrelated to the exercise program.

PROGRESS AND RE-EVALUATE

The program should be progressed at a sensible rate so that the fire fighter continues to make improvements. Re-evaluations should be scheduled frequently to show the fire fighter that his or her hard work is paying off with tangible results. This practice will help maintain motivation and adherence.

GENERAL ADAPTATION SYNDROME

PFTs must take into account the client's ability to adapt to exercise. Hans Selye theorized that the body's response to any stressor follows a distinct pattern he termed the general adaptation syndrome (GAS) (Selye, 1973). The GAS consists of three phases: alarm phase, resistance phase, and exhaustion phase. In the alarm phase, the body responds to a stressor by releasing stress hormones and mobilizing defense mechanisms. When the stressor is the initiation of an exercise program or a new periodization cycle, the alarm phase is marked by a temporary decrease in performance due to soreness or stiffness.

In the adaptation phase, the body attempts to cope with the stressor. When exercise is the stressor, the body initially adapts within two to four weeks by recruiting more motor units, improving coordination between muscle groups, and developing functional motor patterns. Following this initial adaptation period, physiological changes begin to occur (e.g., increase in contractile protein, mitochondria, collateral circulation, muscle glycogen stores, and improved efficiency of energy metabolism). During this phase, the body can begin to adapt to gradual and progressive overloads. An excessive overload during this phase can quickly overwhelm the body's ability to adapt and the recruit may immediately enter into the exhaustion phase.

The exhaustion phase occurs if the stressor (training) is too intense or exists for too great a duration. In this phase, the characteristics of the alarm phase reappear and the desired adaptations are no longer possible. The beginning of this phase is sometimes referred to as over-reaching. If unmanaged, exhaustion can make it difficult for the client to recuperate adequately and lead to overtraining.

OVERLOAD PRINCIPLE

The overload principle states that for an improvement (adaptation) to take place, workloads imposed must exceed those normally encountered. When designing exercise programs, PFTs should base the type and amount of overload on the goals of the program, the experience and fitness level of clients, and each client's ability to recuperate adequately.

Overload can come in many forms. It may be achieved by increasing the amount of weight lifted, the number of repetitions, the speed of movement, the total volume of work performed, the distance run, or the intensity of exertion. Even wearing turnouts or using fire fighting equipment can be adequate to bring about adaptation, especially in recruits. Having a well-designed plan is the key to success.

OVERREACHING AND OVERTRAINING

A good understanding of the overreaching and overtraining phenomena are critical to the success of any fitness program. During overreaching, the client has not fully recuperated from previous workouts or demands before encountering additional overloads. The body must be allowed to obtain active rest when overreaching occurs. Active rest means using several less-demanding workouts (usually around 40% of the maximum effort), and can take two or more weeks to become fully effective. If overreaching is not addressed, the condition worsens and overtraining can occur. This can have long-term detrimental effects on performance as shown in Figure 10.1.

Figure 10.1
Overtraining Syndrome

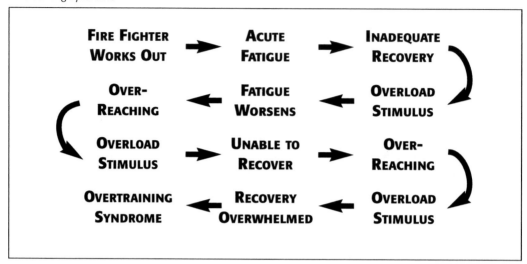

When overtraining occurs, the immune response is greatly diminished, and injury and illness may result. These injuries can be permanent and may alter a client's performance in exercise and activities of daily living for the rest of his or her life. The most reliable sign of overtraining is an increase in the resting pulse of 10 or more beats per minute. Other signs of overtraining include fatigue, muscle soreness, apathy, lack of improvement, lack of appetite, insomnia, and mood swings (Table 10.1).

Table 10.1 Signs of Overtraining

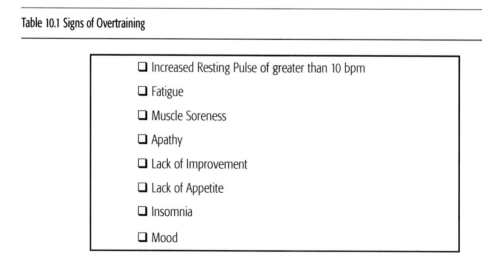

Overtraining requires a long recovery period of several weeks up to one year. During this recovery period, a probationary fire fighter could easily lose motivation to work out, become apathetic about the job, and suffer other illness or injuries. Loss of motivation or additional injuries during this period can be detrimental in motivating these new fire fighters to enjoy lifelong commitment to exercise and wellness. Exercisers that miss more than three successive workouts have a significantly greater chance of dropping out of their fitness program.

One of the keys to preventing overtraining is providing adequate rest. This is one of the greatest challenges during recruit training. As with rest following overreaching, active rest is most effective. During active rest, the recruit continues to exercise but the volume and resistance is significantly decreased. Active rest improves blood flow and can improve the client's ability to recover fully. A second key to prevent overtraining is proper nutrition. The consumption of adequate calories and nutrients is critical to the body's ability to recuperate.

FITT PROGRAMMING

The FITT principle is an easy way to remember the components necessary in a complete fitness program. FITT is a programming model that is appropriate for all aspects of fitness: strength training, cardiovascular training, and flexibility training, and is appropriate for all ages and special populations. The FITT principle incorporates the four variables that must be managed when developing any individualized exercise program, as shown in Table 10.2. Tables 10.3 through 10.5 show ACSM guidelines on cardiovascular, strength, and flexibility training using the FITT principle when programming for healthy adults. Table 10.6 shows ACSM, CDC, and Surgeon General recommendations for programming for highly de-conditioned adults.

Table 10.2   The FITT Principle

F	Frequency – How often is the exercise or activity to be performed in terms of times per day and/or days per week?
I	Intensity – The level of exercise in terms of heart rate, perceived exertion, pounds, strength levels, METS, etc.
T	Time – The duration of the exercise or activity in minutes and/or sets.
T	Type – The mode or description of the exercise or activity.

Adapted from American College of Sports Medicine. (2006). *ACSM's Guidelines for Exercise Testing and Prescription*, 7/e. Philadelphia: Lippincott, Williams & Wilkins.

Table 10.3   ACSM Guidelines for Cardiorespiratory Fitness for Healthy Adults

F	3–5 times per week
I	55–90% of maximum heart rate, perceived exertion "somewhat hard to hard," 40–85% of heart rate reserve or oxygen uptake reserve (VO₂R)
T	20–60 minutes of continuous or intermittent (minimum 10-minute bouts) of aerobic activity accumulated during the day
T	Large muscle groups, rhythmic and aerobic in nature

Adapted from American College of Sports Medicine. (2006). *ACSM's Guidelines for Exercise Testing and Prescription*, 7/e. Philadelphia: Lippincott, Williams & Wilkins.

Table 10.4   ACSM Guidelines for Strength Training for Healthy Adults

F	2–3 times per week
I	At least moderate intensity. Intensity levels should continue to increase to levels above those normally experienced.
T	1 set, 8–12 repetitions for healthy participants under 50 years old 1 set, 10–15 repetitions for participants older than 50 12–20 repetitions for endurance 8–12 repetitions for hypertrophy or size increase 1–8 reps for strength/power
T	Dynamic types of exercises, using full range of motion

Adapted from American College of Sports Medicine. (2006). *ACSM's Guidelines for Exercise Testing and Prescription,* 7/e. Philadelphia: Lippincott, Williams & Wilkins.

Table 10.5   ACSM Guidelines for Flexibility for Healthy Adults

F	A minimum of 2–3 times a week; ideal 5–7 times a week
I	To a position of mild discomfort
T	15–30 seconds for static; 6-second contraction followed by 10–30 seconds assisted stretch for PNF
T	Various techniques including static, dynamic, and PNF for each major muscle and/or tendon group

Adapted from American College of Sports Medicine. (2006). *ACSM's Guidelines for Exercise Testing and Prescription,* 7/e. Philadelphia: Lippincott, Williams & Wilkins.

Table 10.6   ACSM, CDC, and Surgeon General Recommendations for Highly De-conditioned Adults

F	Most days of the week
I	Perceived exertion "moderate," at least 55–64% maximum heart rate
T	30 minutes of activity (minimum 10-minute bouts) accumulated throughout the day
T	Continuous movement or activity including gardening, housework, and other activities of daily living

Adapted from American College of Sports Medicine. (2006). *ACSM's Guidelines for Exercise Testing and Prescription,* 7/e. Philadelphia: Lippincott, Williams & Wilkins.

PROGRESSION

When and how should the FITT program be changed?

❑ Change only one of the FITT components at a time.

❑ Initial *adaptation* to exercise occurs within four to six weeks.

❑ Significant *improvement* usually continues for 12 to 20 weeks.

Maintenance begins when improvement tapers or plateaus, usually about six months after program starts.

FITNESS PROGRAMS FOR RECRUITS

In principle, putting together fitness programs for recruits appears simple. Recruits are motivated to adhere to their programs, have the time and facilities to work out, and usually have 12 to 16 weeks to train. In reality, designing fitness programs for recruits is more complex.

Overtraining may result from the combination of high motivation level of the recruits, high (and sometimes unrealistic) expectations, lack of knowledge of exercise principles by the recruit training officers, high total volume of work performed by the recruits, low initial fitness levels at the time of entry of some recruits, finite length of the training academy program, and peer pressure to perform. Recruits may enter the academy already overtrained after long intense preparatory training programs. In addition, at the start of the academy recruits must adapt to many changes, including the new social environment, pressure to succeed, early and often long hours, and many new physical challenges. Adjustment to these changes can diminish the recruit's ability to recover from the physical, emotional, and mental demands of the training academy.

Recruit fitness programs should include the following:

♦ Introducing the Wellness-Fitness Initiative

♦ Improving recruit fitness and performance

♦ Teaching recruits about how and why to maintain fitness

♦ Teaching injury prevention strategies

Success of recruit fitness programs depend on fire department and recruit training officer support. This support sends the message to recruits that physical fitness is not only important in the academy but also is part of the culture of the department. Support for recruit training can be demonstrated in many ways, including:

♦ Adequate and consistent time to workout

♦ Adequate and safe exercise equipment

♦ Participation in the program by the recruit training officers

♦ The use of PFTs to implement the program

♦ Accurate and dynamic lectures on all aspects of nutrition and fitness

RECRUIT PROGRAM DESIGN

There are numerous ways to build successful recruit fitness programs. As long as the basic exercise principles (i.e., specificity of training, overload principle, law of progression, general adaptation syndrome) are followed and overtraining is prevented, most programs will be successful. Consider the following factors when designing your recruit fitness program:

- Length of the academy
- Number of recruits in the academy
- Amount of time allotted to fitness each day
- Number of days allotted to fitness
- Expertise and availability of PFTs
- Expertise of the recruit training officers
- Amount and type of equipment available
- Demands of the academy
- Experience and fitness of the recruits
- Metabolic, muscular, cardiovascular, and flexibility requirements of the academy

Many different types of fitness programs have been shown to accomplish the goal of safe progressive fitness improvement. One of the most efficient and effective program designs is circuit training. Circuit training allows PFTs to train multiple recruits while using skills similar to those of fire fighting. Circuits can be designed to include weight equipment, body weight exercises, calisthenics, and cardiovascular stations. Variables that can be adjusted progressively include the number of exercises, the time or repetitions completed per station, the rest intervals between exercises, the resistance, the speed of movement, and the total time or number of sets on the circuit. Table 10.7 includes guidelines for recruit training program design.

Table 10.7   Recruit Fitness Training Program Suggestions

☑ Start with slow movements to build safe form and correct motor patterns.
☑ Start with slow aerobic runs to build aerobic base.
☑ Progressively increase total volume with low intensity to build muscular endurance base.
☑ Integrate interval training into cardiovascular training routines.
☑ Increase the volume of circuit training.
☑ Progress circuits by including more exercises.
☑ As fitness levels increase, include anaerobic activities (e.g., stairs, sprints, resistance running).
☑ Increase weight loads to stimulate muscular strength improvements.
☑ Add speed/strength exercises to develop muscular power.
☑ Consider one week of active rest every six to eight weeks to avoid overtraining.
☑ Have recruits take and record their resting pulse every day upon waking.
☑ Have PFTs meet with recruit training officers frequently to adjust programs as needed.
☑ Include a progressive skill course that includes actual fire fighting skills (e.g., forcible entry, hose drag, rescue, search, stair climb, ceiling pull) performed in full turnouts while breathing air.

SUMMARY

Ultimately, the PFTs must remember that the goal of the academy is to train recruits for successful fire fighting careers, not train them for world-class athletic competition. By following sound exercise science, recruits will improve their fitness levels, avoid injuries, and acquire proper fire fighter skills. Historically, it was thought that a recruit graduating the academy must be in the best shape of their career and would invariably deteriorate thereafter. Recruits can continue to improve their conditioning well beyond the training academy in departments that implement the Wellness-Fitness Initiative, use PFTs, and create a culture that supports and encourages physical fitness.

EXERCISE AND PREGNANCY UPDATE

Research has shown that exercise during pregnancy is not only safe, but also beneficial to the health of mother and child. Gone is the belief that a pregnant woman must "baby" herself when it comes to being active and staying physically fit. In 1994, and again in 2002, the American College of Obstetricians and Gynecologists revised its guidelines for exercise during pregnancy (ACOG, 1994 & 2002; http://www.acog.org). Pregnant women should be encouraged to exercise with physician approval. Due to the lack of information, or outdated information, it is inherent that all fitness professionals, especially PFTs, share the updated guidelines with their pregnant clients as shown in Table 10.8.

Table 10.8   Guidelines for Exercising during Pregnancy

Outdated Guidelines	Current Guideline
Exercising during pregnancy causes low birth weight babies.	Research has shown that exercising females have leaner babies.
Exercising heart rate should never exceed 140 beats per minute.	Blanket statements are inappropriate for the variety of fitness levels. Pregnant women are now encouraged to gauge their own fitness levels but not exercise to exhaustion.
Vigorous exercise may lead to a miscarriage.	Studies have shown that the incidence of miscarriage and birth defects is consistent in both non-exercisers and exercisers.
Previously sedentary women should not start an exercise program during pregnancy.	It is now considered safe and highly recommended for a sedentary woman, with medical clearance, to begin exercise programs during pregnancy as long as activity is increased gradually.

AVOID SUPINE POSITION

After the first trimester, while in the supine position, the enlarging uterus can compress the vena cava, the major vein that runs up the back side of the abdomen. As a result, less blood flows back to the heart, potentially decreasing the blood supply to the fetus.

Diastasis, or separation of the rectus abdominis muscle, is also a risk after the first trimester. Performing supine exercises increases the risk of diastasis. However, abdominal muscles should still be worked during pregnancy. Strong abs, especially the transverse abdominals, are crucial during labor. Alternatives to supine exercises include core stabilization exercises and "baby hugs," performed by sitting or standing with shoulders relaxed and contracting abdominal muscles, pulling in the navel as close to the spine as possible.

RELAXIN, THE PREGNANCY HORMONE

Joints and ligaments become more relaxed during pregnancy due to a hormone called relaxin, which also relaxes the pelvic girdle during labor and delivery. All of the joints in the pregnant body are affected and significant concentrations of relaxin can remain in the female's body for six weeks or more postpartum. Therefore, care must be taken to avoid an injury during workouts, especially when performing stretching exercises. Movements that place any joint at risk should be avoided completely. PFTs should keep all movements within a conservative range of motion, and show safe modifications to any questionable exercises or stretches.

DRINK UP: DEHYDRATION IS A RISK

Extra emphasis should be placed on hydration when pregnant, as dehydration can cause premature labor, stress the kidneys, and diminish perspiration. Pregnant women should drink at least 6 to 8 ounces of water every 10 minutes during exercise, consuming no less than 16 to 32 ounces during an hour-long session and the same amount after exercising. Continual and liberal intake of appropriate fluids throughout the day is essential.

Pregnancy impacts how a woman feels during a workout. Some of the most common complaints of pregnant exercisers include shortness of breath, fatigue, nausea, joint and/or ligament discomfort, and a perceived loss of coordination. The new weight distribution may make pregnant women feel more unstable and uncoordinated during activity. These are all normal symptoms resulting from the physical changes that occur during pregnancy. For example, shortness of breath results from heart working harder to boost cardiac output due to increased blood volume. Hormones also contribute to the fatigue and nausea experienced by some women.

Pregnant women require an additional 300 calories per day – possibly more if they exercise regularly. It is recommended that moderate amounts of food be eaten about two hours before exercising and immediately following the workout. Carbohydrates are the best source of energy.

A workout program for a pregnant woman should look very similar in design to that of the non-pregnant exerciser. The workout starts with thorough warm-up, then continues with cardiovascular training, muscle conditioning, and a cool-down stretch. The warm-up should focus on getting the body prepared for the workout by increasing muscle temperature and lubricating the joints. This can be done through the use of simple, low-impact, low-intensity movements or even by spending a few minutes on a cardiovascular machine such as a treadmill or stationary bike. Warm-up movements should include both upper- and lower-body components. The cardiovascular portion of a pregnancy workout should last approximately 20 to 30 minutes or as energy level permits. Cardiovascular machines also have options for increasing intensity without increasing impact. For example, the treadmill can be set on a higher grade or a stair climber can be set on a faster speed. Pregnant women may adhere better to non-impact activities such as cycling and water exercises.

Muscular conditioning is beneficial in preparing the female body for labor and delivery. A variety of equipment can be used as long as the growing abdominal region can be accommodated. Deep squats and max lifts should be avoided. Lunges are only recommended for pregnant women who are experienced weight lifters, who must still use caution due to the extra weight in the mid-section and the potential for loss of balance. Focus on the adductors, abductors, gluteals, and hamstrings; these require extra attention in preparation for labor and delivery. Surprisingly, the upper-body muscles, including the rhomboids, trapezius, and deltoids, also get quite a workout during labor and should not be neglected during a workout. Muscle conditioning should also include moderate abdominal work and Kegel exercises. Kegel exercises will help retain bladder control and assist with the strenuous acts of labor and delivery.

A cool-down is essential to lower the body's core temperature. It should consist of low-intensity, low-impact, and simple movements that give the client adequate time to breathe comfortably. Each workout session should end with at least five minutes of flexibility training and relaxation. Remind women who are extremely flexible not to go beyond their normal range of motion even though the relaxin effect may allow for greater movement.

In summary, the majority of pregnant women can and should exercise even if they were previously inactive. Exercise makes the pregnancy more comfortable and speeds postpartum recovery. Even short periods of activity are beneficial, but regular and consistent exercise is preferred.

It is highly recommended that fire fighters who become pregnant immediately be put on light or restricted duty. Although pregnant fire fighters may be physically capable of performing the tasks of the job, the risk of exposure and injury makes it prudent to reassign the fire fighter during pregnancy.

THE ACOG GUIDELINES

1. Mild to moderate exercise can be continued throughout pregnancy. Regular exercise (three times per week) is preferable to intermittent activity.

2. Exercise in the supine position should be avoided after the first trimester. Vigorous exercise and prolonged periods of motionless standing should be avoided throughout pregnancy.

3. Exercise during pregnancy should be modified according to maternal symptoms – such as lightheadedness, shortness of breath, dizziness, nausea, and fatigue – and may, in some circumstances, be continued at intensity levels similar to those prior to pregnancy. The latest guidelines give women the green light to elevate their heart rate beyond 140 beats per minute and work the abdominal muscles.

4. It is crucial to pay attention to maternal symptoms. Pregnant woman should stop exercising when fatigued and must not exercise to exhaustion.

5. Any type of exercise involving the potential for even mild abdominal trauma should be avoided.

6. Pregnant women require an additional 300 calories per day – possibly more if they exercise regularly.

7. Pregnant exercisers must have adequate hydration, wear appropriate clothing (comfortable, loose-fitting, and breathable) and exercise in optimal environments (with adequate cooling and ventilation).

8. Many of the physiological changes of pregnancy persist for four to six weeks postpartum. Pre-pregnancy exercise routines should be resumed gradually. Physician approval is necessary before resuming exercise programs.

Source: American College of Obstetricians and Gynecologists. (1994). *Exercise During Pregnancy and the Post Partum Period.* ACOG Technical Bulletin, 189.

Table 10.9   FITT Principle for Pregnant Clients

F	2–3 times per week. Regular exercise is better than intermittent. With physician permission, non-exercisers can begin exercise programs as energy level permits. Women who previously exercised can continue their normal exercise program as tolerated.	
I	Mild to moderate intensity, Never to exhaustion Warm up at RPE 2–3 on 1–10 scale, perform cardio at RPE 4–8, or as tolerated	
T	As tolerated depending on prior fitness level, energy level and symptoms 20–30 minutes	
T	Most types of exercise are acceptable, but low- to non-impact is best. Use common sense and caution. Avoid any activity that has the potential for even mild abdominal trauma. Avoid exercise in the supine position after the first trimester.	
S	Avoid intense flexibility training due to laxity in the joints. Avoid exercises that require high levels of balance or require sudden burst of movement.	

Note: S = special considerations

Adapted from American College of Sports Medicine. (2006). *ACSM's Guidelines for Exercise Testing and Prescription,* 7/e. Philadelphia: Lippincott, Williams & Wilkins.

OTHER SPECIAL POPULATIONS

Who is considered to be a part of the group termed *special populations*? We typically think of special populations as being made up of individuals with disabilities. In reality, special populations include all individuals who are part of the larger continuum of exercising individuals but are not typically described as healthy adults. Special populations include clients falling into one or more of the following categories: pregnancy, hypertension, coronary artery disease, diabetes, asthma, and obesity. Age (adolescents and seniors), arthritis, and low-back pain also require special considerations.

The physiological benefits of training and relative improvement are seen in almost all adults. When designing fitness programs for special populations, an additional component to the FITT principle is S, for special considerations. Considerations for special populations are discussed below and summarized in Tables 10.10 through 10.16.

CORONARY ARTERY DISEASE

Clients with coronary artery disease (CAD) *must* obtain release from a Fire Department physician, have completed at least the Phase II Cardiac rehab program, and have a functional capacity of 6 to 8 METS. A cardiologist or other designated health professional must provide the PFT with an upper-limit heart rate, as well as guidelines and limitations to physical activity.

(Refer to the *ACE Personal Trainer Manual* pages 346 to 347 for more information.)

Table 10.10   FITT Principle for Clients with Coronary Artery Disease

F	Depending on fatigue, 3–7 days per week, 2 times per day with short sessions
I	Moderate, RPE of 9–14 on scale of 6–20, 40% of VO$_2$ max, peak exercise intensity should be about 10 bpm under the HR that elicits signs/symptoms
T	Start with 10 minutes per session not including warm-up and cool-down. Increase every 1–3 weeks, as tolerated, up to 30–60 minute sessions.
T	Aerobic Endurance: walking, bicycling, swimming, etc.
	Muscular Endurance: low intensity, range of motion
S	Special Considerations: Extended warm-up and cool-down, avoid isometric exercises, avoid Valsalva maneuver, as it increases blood pressure. Dietary and lifestyle adjustments may be necessary

HYPERTENSION

Hypertension is defined as a blood pressure over 140/90. Clients can only work out after blood pressure is brought under control and they have obtained a physician approval.

(Refer to the *ACE Personal Trainer Manual* pages 347 to 349 for more information.)

Table 10.11 FITT Principle for Clients with Hypertension

F	3–7 times per week. Short, more frequent sessions are preferred over longer, less frequent sessions
I	Aerobic Training: RPE low to moderate, 40–70% max HR Strength Training: low intensity with higher repetitions (12–20). Avoid Valsalva maneuver, isometrics, and high intensity
T	Begin with short intermittent sessions, then gradually increase to 30–60 minutes
T	Aerobic Endurance: walking, swimming, bicycling, etc. Muscular Endurance: circuit training, low intensity
S	Special Considerations: Extended warm-up and cool-down. Resistance training by itself may not lower resting BP. Lifestyle adjustments necessary (e.g., lower consumption of alcohol, smoking cessation, lower salt intake, stress management, cholesterol reduction). If client's blood pressure is above 140/90 on at least two different occasions, suggest that he or she see a physician.

OBESITY

Obesity is defined as women having over 30% body fat and men as having over 25% body fat. As with all special populations, physician approval is required.

(Refer to the *ACE Personal Trainer Manual* pages 362 to 363 for more information. See also the National Institutes of Health Web site at www.nih.gov.)

Table 10.12 FITT Principle for Clients with Obesity

F	Minimum 5 days a week, but 7 days a week is optimum
I	Start with low-to-moderate intensity, 40 to 50% max HR, RPE 4–7 Work up to 50–60% max HR, RPE 10–13 Strength Training: 8–12 repetitions, 1–2 sets
T	40–60 minute sessions or multiple shorter sessions of 20–30 minutes per day, if longer sessions can not be tolerated. If intensity must be lowered, extend time to 60–120 minutes. Total time should be long enough to burn at least 300–500 calories per session and at least a weekly total of 2500 kcal.
T	Low- or non-impact endurance: swimming, walking, bicycling, etc. Weightbearing activities might not be tolerated due to joint discomfort. Muscular Strength: goal is to increase muscle mass
S	Special Considerations: Encourage activities that are enjoyable. Referral to nutritionist and set goals for gradual, sustained weight loss (1–2 lbs. per week;10% from baseline over 6 months). Be aware of self-consciousness and body image issues.

Waist circumference is one of the best indicators of health risk associated with body composition for obese clients—defined as waist girth of > 101 cm (40 inches) for men and 89 cm (35 inches) for women.

DIABETES

Diabetes is a disease in which the body does not produce insulin sufficient to meet the demands for glucose metabolism, typically resulting in high blood sugar levels. Type 2 diabetes accounts for 90 to 95% of cases and is related to increased age, obesity, and sedentary lifestyle. Since exercise increases the body's need for glucose, it is important to work with the diabetes client in monitoring blood sugar level closely, especially when starting or modifying exercise. As with all special needs clients, clearance from a physician is required.

(Refer to the *ACE Personal Trainer Manual* pages 351 to 353 for more information. See also the American Diabetes Association Web site at http://www.diabetes.org and the Canadian Diabetes Association at http://www.diabetes.ca/.)

Table 10.13 FITT Principle for Clients with Diabetes

	Type 1	Type 2
Insulin	Insulin dependent, must take injections	Non-insulin dependent, takes oral medications
Genetic	No	Yes
Percent of Diabetics	10%	90%
Age	Younger	Adult-Onset/Younger Obese
Weight	Normal	Overweight

F	4–6 days/week, or daily at lower intensity	High frequency to encourage weight loss, 4-7 times per week
I	50–85% VO₂max 60–90% HRmax	Low intensity preferred Start with RPE 11–13, 40–50% VO₂ max Work up to RPE 12–15, 50–85% VO₂ max
T	20–30 minutes	Long duration, work up to 40–60 minutes
T	Endurance	Endurance
S	Special Considerations: Avoid injecting insulin in muscles to be used in exercise session. Strive for consistency in exercise regime.	Special Considerations: May have sensitive feet due to poor circulation. Clients using sulfonylureas should consume extra carbohydrates with exercise.

ASTHMA

Asthma is a respiratory disease in which a variety of factors (dust, chemicals, exercise) trigger narrowing of the airways by smooth muscle contraction and inflammation of the cells lining the airway. An asthmatic reaction is characterized by labored breathing, often with audible wheezing. Review medication plans with clients with asthma and specific triggers. Keep in mind that overexertion, especially in cold air, may trigger symptoms.

(Refer to the *ACE Personal Trainer Manual* pages 353 to 354, the American Lung Association at www.lungusa.org, and the Canadian Lung Association at www.lung.ca for more information.)

Table 10.14   FITT Principle for Clients with Asthma

F	At least 3–4 times per week.
I	Intensity based on client's fitness level and level of tolerance
T	Work up to 20–45 minutes. If functional capacity is low, 10 minute sessions, 2 or 3 times per day
T	Endurance-type activities
S	Special Considerations: Extended warm-up and cool-down. Keep inhaler available during exercise sessions

OSTEOARTHRITIS

Osteoarthritis is a joint disease characterized by loss of cartilage at the affected joints. Since cartilage cushions the joints, cartilage loss results in bones rubbing against each other causing inflammation, pain, and loss of movement. Obesity and previous joint injuries are risk factors for osteoarthritis. Exercise emphasizing flexibility and muscle strength are essential to relieving pain and increasing joint flexibility.

(Refer to the *ACE Personal Trainer Manual* pages 358 to 360, the Arthritis Foundation at http://www.arthritis.org/, and the Arthritis Society at http://www.arthritis.ca for more information.)

Table 10.15   FITT Principle for Clients with Arthritis

F	5–7 times per week depending on tolerance. Goal of 1500 kcal per week
I	Low-intensity, pain-free movement, minimize stress on joints
T	10–15 minute sessions Progress only if pain free to 30–60 minutes
T	Non-weightbearing activities (e.g., cycling, water aerobics, swimming). Warm water exercise is preferred
S	Special Considerations: Avoid isometrics due to joint stress. Include exercises that improve balance to reduce risk of falling. If overweight, goals should include reduction of body weight.

YOUTH (CHILDREN AND ADOLESCENTS)

Children are considered a special population due to their immature bodies and minds. The most important thing to remember when developing exercise programs for children is to make the programs enjoyable so that the children will continue to exercise throughout their adulthood.

(Refer to the *ACE Personal Trainer Manual* pages 363 to 365 for more information.)

Table 10.16 FITT Principle for Child and Adolescent Clients

	Cardiovascular Training	Strength Training
F	Younger children: Most days of the week accumulate at least 30 minutes of activity Older children: vigorous activity at least 3 times a week	Limit to 2 sessions per week
I	Start slow and progress gradually. Use perceived exertion to monitor intensity	Weight loads should be used that permit 8 or more repetitions. Avoid severe muscle fatigue. Overload by first increasing repetitions, and then weight if appropriate. Avoid repetitive use of heavy weights until reaching Tanner stage 5 (adolescence) level of developmental maturity
T	Work up to at least 30 minutes	1–2 sets of 8–10 different exercises with 8–12 repetitions per set Rest at least 1–2 minutes between exercises
T	A variety of activities that use large muscle groups and weightbearing activities. Encourage a variety of recreational and life-time activities	Use all major muscle groups. Try to alternate muscle groups, as in a "push-pull" routine
S	Provide positive experiences and safe facilities	All strength training activities should be supervised. Promote positive experiences

SUMMARY

General principles of fitness training apply to all programs: consistent regular training is best, clients must be trained to exercise safely and supervised at regular intervals, fitness routines must be varied to promote improvement, and rest periods must be built in to avoid overtraining. Specific approaches to fitness can be modified easily to accommodate client goals and needs. Using the FITT programming structure, PFTs can give clients concrete guidance to ensure that clients clearly understand what they must do to reach their fitness goals.

REFERENCES

American College of Obstetricians ands Gynecologists. (1994). *Exercise During Pregnancy and the Post Partum Period*. ACOG Technical Bulletin, 189.

American College of Obstetricians and Gynecologists. (2002). ACOG Committee Opinion: *Exercise During Pregnancy and the Postpartum Period*. Washington, D.C.: American College of Obstetricians and Gynecologists.

American College of Sports Medicine. (2006). *ACSM's Guidelines for Exercise Testing and Prescription*, 7th ed. Philadelphia: Lippincott, Williams & Wilkins.

Selye, H. (1973). The evolution of the stress concept. *American Scientist*. 61, 692–699.

FIRE FIGHTER– SPECIFIC DISEASES

In many fire departments throughout the U.S. and Canada, PFTs will be considered health experts. PFTs are not experts, as was discussed in the professional responsibility chapter, but they should be familiar with health-related references if a fire fighter comes to them with cancer, heart disease, or an infectious disease that was contracted on the job. The following material was derived from IAFF manuals specific to cancer, heart disease, and infectious diseases. The complete manuals can be obtained from the IAFF Occupational Health and Safety Department.

PFT candidates are not responsible for this information for the purposes of the PFT certification exam.

OCCUPATIONAL CANCER AND THE FIRE SERVICE

Cancer is the second leading cause of death in the United States, exceeded only by heart disease (U.S. Department of Health and Human Services, 1999). It is the leading cause of death for those aged 45 to 64. The American Cancer Society estimates that 555,500 Americans will die of cancer in 2002 and about 1.3 million new cases of cancer will be diagnosed in 2002. Of these deaths, evidence suggests that at least one-third could be prevented by changes in lifestyle factors including obesity and physical inactivity (American Cancer Society – www.cancer.org).

Fire fighters and emergency medical responders often face special occupational risks of cancer due to exposure to potential carcinogens (cancer-causing agents). Cancer in fire fighters has been an area of concern and focus for the International Association of Fire Fighters and others for several decades. Fire fighters and EMS personnel are exposed to a multitude of known carcinogenic chemicals, as well as many other types of chemicals with unknown carcinogenic potential.

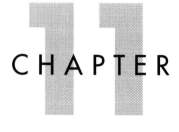

CHAPTER

Although medical progress has lead to improvements in the diagnosis and treatment of cancer, prevention remains the best method of decreasing the number of cancer-related deaths. Identifying cancer-causing agents and avoiding exposure to these agents are key to prevention. In the past 30 years, researchers have identified many agents that cause cancer in humans. Agencies such as the Occupational Safety and Heath Administration (OSHA), the National Institute of Occupational Safety and Health (NIOSH), and the International Agency for Research on Cancer (IARC) have published guidelines for protecting workers and the general population from known carcinogens.

This section contains a review and analysis of several topics, including known carcinogens in fire fighters' environments, types of cancers known to affect fire fighters, and cancer prevention strategies for fire fighters and emergency medical responders. Throughout this section, information and statistics are presented from both Canada and the U.S.

BASIC FACTS ABOUT CANCER

DEFINING CANCER

Cancer is a group of diseases characterized by the uncontrolled growth and spread of abnormal cells. The term cancer defines groups of distinct diseases that share many common characteristics: rapid growth of cells, lack of normal cell differentiation and function, and survival and spread of abnormal cells.

CAUSES OF CANCER

Cancer may be caused by external factors including chemical, physical, and biological agents, as well as internal factors such as hormones, inherited mutations, and immune conditions. Often, many causal factors work together to initiate and promote the development of a cancer. Exposures to certain chemicals in the workplace may take 10 or more years to cause mutations (altered cells) and detectable cancers.

CANCER PREVENTION

All cancers caused by cigarette smoking and heavy use of alcohol can be completely prevented. Lifestyle changes such as smoking cessation and reduction of dietary fat can decrease cancer risk. Screening tests that detect early stages of cancer and precancerous changes can improve cancer survival.

CANCER TREATMENT

Cancer may be treated using surgery, chemotherapy, radiation therapy, immunotherapy, and hormone treatment. Treatment varies depending upon the specific type of cancer and stage (degree of spread). Cancer treatment is a dynamic field, with options changing as new treatments are discovered and investigated. A discussion of the treatment of specific types of cancer is beyond the scope of this text.

TYPES OF CARCINOGENS

Carcinogens are agents that start the cancer process. This section discusses three types of carcinogens: chemicals, viruses, and radiation. Individual susceptibility to those agents is determined by many factors, including age, gender, genetics, frequency of exposure to the agent, and duration of exposure.

Chemicals

Several million chemicals exist and approximately 50,000 chemicals are regularly used in business and industry. It is not known how many of these chemicals used in industry are carcinogenic, but fewer than 1,000 have been tested for carcinogenic activity, since the testing process for identifying carcinogens is expensive and time consuming.

Viruses

Approximately 15% of human cancers may be caused by viruses (Hausen, 1991). This is a relatively new area of investigation in human cancer research, even though viruses have been known to cause cancer in animals since early in this century. Certain viruses have been shown to be associated with specific cancers. Cancer causation by viruses occurs by several different and complex mechanisms. Hepatitis B and C viruses are thought to cause liver cancer through repeated damage to liver cells. The chronic regeneration of liver cells that results from this damage, coupled with accumulation of damage to DNA, eventually results in cancer. Infection with HIV has been associated with development of Kaposi's sarcoma.

Radiation

Radiation is a form of energy. The most hazardous form of radiation is ionizing radiation, which can severely damage cells and tissues. Ionizing radiation is produced naturally through the decay of unstable radioactive elements. During decay, elements change their atomic structure by releasing various types of particles. X-ray machines and other devices can also artificially produce radiation. This process uses large amounts of electricity to generate the radiation.

Fire fighters may encounter ionizing radiation when responding to emergencies at medical offices, hospitals, television repair shops, petroleum refineries, and scientific research laboratories, and at factories that produce medicines, smoke detectors, or X-ray tubes. The level of hazard depends on the particular type of emergency. Experience has shown that workers exposed to radiation have increased rates of occupational illnesses such as cancer, leukemia, sterility, and cataracts (Rom, 1998). In addition, radiation exposure could also affect the unborn fetus of a pregnant fire fighter.

THE FIRE FIGHTING ENVIRONMENT

Health studies of occupational groups continually examine the hazards encountered in the work environment. In the case of fire fighting, the products of combustion are the focus of investigation. Several undisputed human carcinogens have been measured in the fire environment. Combustion and the composition and amount of by-products produced are functions of the source materials as well as the conditions of combustion. These conditions include the amount of oxygen present (the ventilation of the fire) and the thermal energy transferred to the burning materials (Lees, 1995).

Combustion products include thousands of chemical constituents, from the simplest products of water and carbon dioxide (the results of burning wood and natural materials) to the components of burning plastics from furnishings and home products. At the site of wildland fires, fire fighters are exposed to herbicides and fire retardant chemicals (Steenland et al., 1996). Industrial fires are even more complex and the combustion products depend on the component materials used and the processes performed at the site. The ubiquitous use of plastics and other synthetic materials increases the likelihood of hazardous materials in fire smoke, leading to the adage that "a car fire is a hazmat incident."

Environmental hazardous materials incidents present a mixed picture, because the exposure is usually only a few chemicals produced or spilled. However, these chemicals could be released at very high concentrations or in an uncommonly encountered exposure scenario. Fire fighters and other first responders could be exposed to any of the 50,000 or more chemicals in commercial use.

Studies of the Fire Fighting Environment

It is difficult to characterize chemical exposures in the fire-fighting environment due to limits on technically feasible methods to measure and analyze combustion-derived materials. Equipment and methods for detecting chemicals in smoke, which were developed in industrial environments with lower contaminant concentrations, can be overwhelmed on the fire ground. In addition, the nature of a fire scene – unplanned, emergent, and life threatening – hampers information collection. The data that are available come from the few studies where direct measures of exposure have been made and from indirect sources including area sampling at working fires and simulated test burns.

Some well-designed studies have quantified concentrations of specific chemicals in the fire-fighting environment through direct personal sampling of fire fighters or area sampling of working fires. The seventeen chemicals found using these methods have been documented (McDiarmid et al., 1991). A modified list of 10 agents found more commonly or in higher concentrations has been discussed in a subsequent review (Steenland et al., 1996). In contrast to this short list, a very long list of over 90 chemicals can be compiled if presence of a chemical in a fire is the only criterion for inclusion, rather than actual concentration measured (Henriks-Eckerman et al., 1990; Lowry et al., 1985; Atlas et al., 1985).

It is important to note that concentrations of contaminants in the environment are not actual fire fighter exposures. Environmental measurements are made within the breathing zone of the fire fighter, and actual exposures are somewhat less when respiratory protective equipment is properly used. Assuming a protection factor of 2,000 (common for the positive pressure demand-type SCBA most commonly used by fire fighters) actual exposures are probably 2,000 times less than the concentrations reported (Steenland et al., 1996). Short-term higher exposures, perhaps approaching levels in the fire-fighting environment, may occur as a result of temporary misfit of respirators. During the overhaul phase, when respiratory protective equipment is less frequently used, air concentrations of some chemicals may be as high as or higher than those reported during the fire-fighting phase (Burgess et al., 1999; Barnard & Weber, 1979).

FIRE SMOKE

Many homes and public buildings are built and furnished with flammable synthetic materials (i.e., plastics) that give off large amounts of smoke and toxic gases when burned. The composition of smoke varies depending upon the type of fire and local conditions (Guidotti & Clough, 1992). A different set of chemicals in different concentrations exists for every material burned and every set of combustion conditions (Lees, 1995).

The health effects of exposure to fire smoke can be acute (short-term), chronic (long-term), or both. Both acute and chronic effects can be life threatening. It is important to note that similar toxins may be found in smoke present during knockdown as well as during overhaul.

1. Components of fire smoke include irritants and asphyxiants (Bizovi & Leikin, 1995).

2. Irritants cause direct injury to the cells that make up the lining of the respiratory system.

3. Asphyxiants block the oxygen-carrying capacity of the blood, so that less oxygen is delivered to the brain and other organs. Irritation and asphyxiation are acute effects of exposure to fire smoke.

4. Some irritants, including hydrogen chloride (HCl), can be absorbed onto small carbon particles in smoke and be inhaled deeply into the lung tissues, producing damage to these tissues.

    a. Other combustion products may be carcinogenic (Golden et al., 1995).

    b. Benzene is a carcinogen that may be present in fire smoke.

5. Carbon dioxide and carbon monoxide gas are present in virtually all fire fighting environments (Froines et al., 1987). Other components of combustion smoke depend upon the substances being burned. In some cases, fire suppression may result in formation of new toxic agents. For example, a combination of sulfur dioxide and water results in the formation of sulfuric acid, which is a respiratory irritant. Exposure to such secondarily formed agents may be significant during overhaul operations (Froines et al., 1987).

DIESEL EXHAUST

If the diesel engines are routinely started in the firehouse, fire fighters may inhale diesel exhaust (Froines et al., 1987). Diesel exhaust is a complex mixture of particulates and gases. The composition of the mixture varies with fuel and engine type, maintenance, tuning, and exhaust gas treatment. Exhaust gases include carbon dioxide, carbon monoxide, nitric oxide, nitrogen dioxide, oxides of sulfur, and hydrocarbons (formaldehyde, methane, benzene, phenol, acrolein, and polycyclic aromatic hydrocarbons). Exhaust particulates are composed of a solid carbon core with a sticky surface. Polynuclear aromatic hydrocarbons, the most common of the organic polycyclic aromatic hydrocarbons (PAHs), attach themselves to the particle surface. Diesel engines emit at least 10 times more nitrogen-PAHs than gasoline engines (Garshick & Schenker, 1996).

There is conclusive evidence that diesel exhaust is mutagenic and carcinogenic in animals. The International Agency for Research on Cancer (IARC) has classified diesel engine exhaust as a probable human carcinogen, associated with lung and bladder cancer (International Agency for Research on Cancer, 1989). PAHs, specifically nitrogen-PAHs, account for much of the mutagenicity observed (Karstadt, 1998). An increased risk of lung cancer has been found consistently among studies conducted on workers with high exposure to diesel exhaust (Bhatia et al., 1998; McDiarmid et al., 1991). There was no pattern of excess bladder cancer risk seen in these studies (Talaska et al., 1996); however, there was evidence that occupational exposure to diesel fuel or fumes increased the risk of prostate cancer (Gustavsson et al., 1998).

CANCERS ASSOCIATED WITH FIRE FIGHTING

As discussed in the previous section, fire fighters are at increased risk of exposure to certain carcinogens, and are therefore at increased risk of developing certain cancers. Research has conclusively demonstrated that fire fighters have increased incidence of leukemia, multiple myeloma, non-Hodgkin's lymphoma, bladder cancer, and brain cancer compared to other workers (Golden et al., 1995; McDiarmid et al., 1991; Siemiatycki, 1991). Additional research indicates that fire fighters may be at increased risk for prostate, large intestine, and skin cancers. It is likely that better, larger studies will strengthen the link between fire fighting as an occupation and specific cancers.

Studies are likely to undercount cases among fire fighters for several reasons. Fire fighters as a group may be more resistant to disease. Due to the rigorous physical demands of fire fighting, fire fighters may be healthier compared with the general population. Also, fire fighters who become ill may change to other occupations. This "double healthy worker effect" may lead to reduced risk estimates for diseases in fire fighters (Guidotti, 1998). In addition, cancer may be under-reported among fire fighters because many retire at age 50 to 55 and there is a long latency period for several cancers. As a result, fire fighters who are diagnosed with cancer after retirement from the fire service may not be included in these studies.

Many studies of causes of death among fire fighters use death certificate data. However, death certificate information is usually incomplete and may not reflect all cases of cancer. Only the immediate cause of death may be included, and other illnesses, such as cancer, may be omitted. Information on occupation is often not included on death certificates, and if included, may only reflect the current occupation at the time of death. Thus, studies that depend on death certificate information may underestimate the number of cases of cancer in fire fighters.

CANCER PREVENTION

Cancer prevention can be divided into primary prevention and secondary prevention. Primary prevention is aimed at stopping a cancer from developing, and includes avoidance of hazards and behavioral changes to decrease individual risk factors for cancer. Secondary prevention includes techniques that detect early cancer or precancerous conditions so that early interventions can decrease the risk of advanced disease. Screening tests are examples of secondary prevention. This section describes several screening tests for cancers more often seen in fire fighters.

PERSONAL PROTECTIVE EQUIPMENT

Fire fighters are exposed to a variety of airborne contaminants, including particulate smoke. As discussed previously, diesel exhaust contains many chemicals, including PAHs, which are known carcinogens. Use of appropriate personal protective equipment (i.e., self-contained breathing apparatus) during fire fighting and overhaul activities decreases exposure to airborne contaminants. Consistent use of universal precautions (e.g., gloves, masks) decreases exposure to blood-borne pathogens such as hepatitis B, hepatitis C, and human immunodeficiency virus (HIV). Personal protective equipment must be maintained in good operating condition to provide the highest level of protection.

DIESEL EXHAUST CONTROL DEVICES

Diesel exhaust is pervasive in the fire fighter's environment, both at the fire station and at the fire scene. The best method to reduce fire fighter exposure to diesel exhaust is installation and use of engineering controls. Diesel exhaust control devices connect to the tail pipes of apparatus and transport exhaust fumes to the exterior of the building, and away from the indoor air supply of the fire station. Other practices that can reduce exposure include isolation of living quarters from the engine room, reduction of exhaust emissions through regular maintenance of engines, use of exhaust fans or smoke ejectors to move fumes away from living quarters, regular cleaning of living quarters, including draperies, and storage of safety clothing away from direct contact with diesel fumes (Girod, 1990).

TOBACCO AND CANCER

All cancers caused by cigarette smoking can be prevented. Despite the large amount of money and recent nationwide focus to prevent smoking and encourage smoking cessation, smoking remains a significant cause of human cancer. In women, lung cancer has recently overtaken breast cancer as the leading cause of cancer deaths.

People who smoke are 10 times more likely to develop lung cancer than nonsmokers. Smokers are likewise more prone to develop cancers of the throat, mouth, esophagus, pancreas, and bladder. Smoking alone accounts for a significant amount of disease and death. What is particularly important for fire fighters is that smoking strongly increases the carcinogenic impact of other chemicals on the human body.

Workers who smoke and are exposed to asbestos have a greatly increased risk of bronchogenic lung cancer. The risk of cancer deaths in workers who smoke and are exposed to asbestos is much higher than that of workers with occupational exposure to asbestos alone. The risk of cancer for workers exposed to rubber or fluorocarbon polymer fumes, chlorine, and carbon dust is also significantly higher in workers who smoke. The Wellness-Fitness Initiative recommends that fire departments only hire new fire fighters who do not smoke, and prohibit them from smoking for the duration of their career.

SMOKING CESSATION

Studies have shown that five years after quitting smoking, the risk of developing cancer of the mouth, throat, and esophagus is half that of a current smoker. Ten years after quitting smoking, the risk of developing lung cancer falls to half that of a smoker, and the risk of cancer of the bladder, kidney, and pancreas significantly decreases (Centers for Disease Control and Prevention, 1990).

The IAFF has published *The IAFF Smoking Cessation Manual: Issues, Policies, and Programs* to assist in smoking cessation efforts. It outlines the most commonly used techniques, including aversive therapy, self-help and group programs, nicotine replacement (patches or gum), acupuncture, and other methods. The Wellness-Fitness Initiative recommends that fire departments provide smoking cessation programs to incumbent fire fighters.

If you desire additional information on individual smoking cessation programs or if your department wishes to begin a smoking cessation program, contact the IAFF Department of Occupational Health and Safety.

USE OF ALCOHOL

When death rates are compared among heavy drinkers (three+ drinks/day) to those who drink moderate amounts of alcohol (one to two drinks/day), studies have shown that heavy drinkers may be at greater risk of dying from certain cancers. Heavy drinking of alcoholic beverages increases the risk of cancers of the esophagus, mouth, throat, larynx, and liver. The risk of getting cancer is magnified when a person combines heavy drinking and smoking. The American Cancer Society estimates that 19,000 cancer deaths in 2002 will be related to excessive alcohol use often in conjunction with tobacco use.

DIET

There is a great deal of research and information concerning the connection between dietary behaviors and cancer. Researchers have estimated that dietary modification could reduce the incidence of fatal cancers by approximately 35% (Doll & Peto, 1981). A diet that is high in saturated fat may lead to increased incidence of cancer of the colon and breast. There are many dietary factors that can affect cancer risk, including type of foods eaten, food preparation methods, portion sizes, food variety, and caloric intake. In general, eating a balanced diet containing the appropriate number of calories and a variety of foods will ensure proper nutrition. Studies are still currently investigating the role of particular nutrients in decreasing cancer risk.

The American Cancer Society Guidelines on Diet, Nutrition, and Cancer Prevention

1. Choose most of the foods you eat from plant sources:
   - Eat five or more servings of fruits and vegetables each day.
   - Eat other foods from plant sources, such as breads, cereals, grain products, rice, pasta, and beans, several times each day.

2. Limit your intake of high-fat foods, particularly from animal sources:
   - Choose foods low in fat.
   - Limit consumption of meats, especially high-fat meats.

3. Be physically active; achieve and maintain a healthy weight:
   - Be at least moderately active for 30 minutes or more on most days of the week.
   - Stay within your healthy weight range.

4. Limit consumption of alcoholic beverages, if you drink at all.

The Wellness-Fitness Initiative includes a diet and nutrition component as well as a program to encourage regular physical activity and maintenance of a healthy weight.

EXPOSURE TO IONIZING RADIATION

In the course of performing their duties, fire fighters spend a considerable amount of time working outdoors. Limiting exposure to ultraviolet radiation by consistent use of sunscreen protection can prevent skin cancer. Use of a sunscreen with sun protection factor (SPF) of 15 or more is recommended (American Cancer Society, 1993). In addition, sunscreen should be used during outdoor activities when off duty.

SCREENING

Early detection of cancer or precancerous conditions through screening tests allows prompt treatment to decrease the severity of disease and increase the chances of survival. Recommendations for screening tests vary by age, gender, and other risk factors for cancer. The Wellness-Fitness Initiative recommends screening for possible occupation-related diseases in fire fighters. Some examples of screening tests and their corresponding cancers are given in Table 11.1.

SUMMARY

Cancer prevention includes decreasing the risk of cancer through changing lifestyle behaviors, avoiding hazards, and detecting and treating cancers in early stages. Many of the lifestyle behavior changes discussed above will also result in decreased risks of non-cancerous conditions, such as heart disease and improved overall health and well being. As research identifies more risk-reduction strategies, cancer prevention may expand to include medical recommendations for dietary or hormonal supplements.

Table 11.1 Cancer Screening Tests

Test	Cancer
Papanicolou (Pap) smear	Cervical dysplasia, cervical cancer
Mammogram	Breast cancer
Prostate specific antigen blood test (PSA)	Prostate cancer
Digital rectal exam	Prostate cancer
Fecal occult blood test	Colon cancer
Colonoscopy	Colon Cancer

OCCUPATIONAL HEART DISEASE AND FIRE FIGHTERS

From before birth until death, the heart performs as a pump, forcing blood through the circulatory system without interruption. Without this function, serious brain damage can occur within 4 to 5 minutes and certain death within 10 minutes. Heart disease is the major killer of both men and women in the United States and Canada. Clearly, the importance of a healthy heart cannot be overstated.

Heart disease can be prevented and treated. Increased social awareness of the adverse health effects of a high fat diet, smoking, obesity, and sedentary lifestyle has changed the way many people care for themselves. The result of "healthier" lifestyles, as well as improving treatments for heart disease, has been a decrease in the death rate from heart attacks over the past two decades.

The section contains a review and an analysis of several topics, including the evidence that fire fighters and emergency medical responders are at increased risk for developing heart disease, the normal anatomy and function of the heart, the types of diseases that afflict the heart, the factors that increase fire fighters' risk of developing heart disease, and what fire fighters and emergency medical responders can do to prevent heart disease.

Throughout this section, information and statistics are presented from both Canada and the United States. While specific numbers differ between the two countries, the trends are nearly identical and could be readily interchanged.

REVIEW OF FIRE FIGHTER MORTALITY STUDIES

Fire fighters have voiced concern that they have unusually high rates of heart disease. One of the few ways to assess the validity of this concern is to analyze heart disease rates in fire fighter mortality studies.

Mortality studies look at the number of deaths in a group, such as fire fighters, to determine if a particular disease is causing more deaths than expected. Many mortality studies of fire fighters have been performed, looking for an association between fire fighting and various diseases. The results have been mixed.

Problems with Mortality Studies

Most mortality studies gather information using death certificates of former fire fighters. The number of deaths in fire fighters due to various causes is compared to another group, the reference population, to look for differences. A typical comparison group is the overall United States' white male population. However, this is not the most appropriate comparison group. There are important differences between fire fighters and this reference group, other than the experience of fire fighting. In general, qualified fire service personnel are healthier than the rest of the U.S. population. Ideally, the study and comparison groups would have similar race, gender, age, health index, and lifestyle profiles, and the profession of fire fighting would be the only significant difference. In reality, some differences will exist, leaving the results of such studies open to interpretation and debate.

Mortality studies also rely on accurate coding of death certificates. However, the diagnostic categories used are general and often overlap, adding uncertainty to the studies. In comparison with cancer, cardiovascular disease is not very accurately diagnosed and recorded on death certificates. For example, one doctor may classify a death as a "heart attack" while a different doctor may classify the same death as "sudden death due to arrhythmia." Both doctors may have made accurate (and related) diagnoses, but the current death certificate system may not reconcile the differences and similarities of these diagnoses. As a result, one diagnosis may be counted as a death due to atherosclerotic coronary vascular disease, while the other might not be.

Another source of uncertainty arises if a fire fighter leaves the job because of cardiovascular disease, or if a fire fighter develops heart disease but dies from another cause, such as cancer or an accident. Many fire fighters can no longer work as fire fighters after they develop cardiovascular disease. These cases would not be counted in mortality studies, and therefore mortality studies may tend to underestimate the risk of cardiovascular disease. Remember, these studies actually measure the risk of *death* from cardiovascular disease, rather than the risk of *developing* cardiovascular disease.

Studies of fire fighters also suffer a limitation known as the "healthy worker effect." In part, fire fighters are selected for employment on the basis of their physical fitness. They are in fact healthier than the general population because less healthy individuals are less likely to be hired as fire fighters. Because of this selection bias, fire fighters would be expected to have a decreased incidence of cardiovascular disease mortality when compared to the general population. Therefore, it would take a very large increase in fire fighter cardiovascular mortality to result in a significant measurable increase in a mortality study.

Between individual fire fighters, the types and amounts of toxic exposure vary from fire to fire and job to job. In addition, lifetime exposure can vary considerably with the use, or lack of use, of personal protective equipment. Because accurate data about hazardous exposures is not available, researchers commonly lump all fire fighters together for study and duration of employment is generally used as a substitute for dose. These study techniques may dilute a real effect from a particular exposure that affects only a portion of fire fighters. Despite the problems associated with mortality studies and the tendency for any real effects to be obscured, several studies have reported an increased risk of cardiovascular disease in fire fighters.

HEART DISEASE

The function of the heart can be divided into several systems that all act in concert to ensure normal function. Each of these systems is prone to specific problems, which can disrupt the overall function of the heart. Furthermore, abnormal function (dysfunction) in any one system may result in abnormal function in a different system.

The complexities of the heart and heart disease have filled many medical textbooks. The purpose of this section is to review the more common diseases that afflict the heart. Each subsection will discuss the diseases that primarily affect a specific heart system.

DISEASES OF THE CORONARY ARTERIES

The coronary arteries provide the myocardium with the oxygen and nutrients needed to maintain normal function. A number of disease processes can interrupt the flow of blood through these arteries, resulting in different kinds of health problems. The most common problem is blockage of the coronary arteries by cholesterol plaques, a disease process called atherosclerosis.

Atherosclerosis

Athero is the Greek term for "gruel" and refers to the cholesterol deposits that build up in the arteries. *Sclerosis* is the Greek term for "hardness" and refers to the hard nature of the cholesterol plaques in arteries. Atherosclerosis is a disease process causing thickening and hardening of the medium and large sized arteries. It is the underlying cause of the vast majority of the heart attacks and strokes that occur in the United States and Canada.

When atherosclerotic plaques build up and sufficiently block the flow of blood in the coronary arteries and cause symptoms, all the different resulting diseases are collectively called atherosclerotic coronary vascular disease (ASCVD) or atherosclerotic heart disease (ASHD). Many authors simply refer to this process by the less precise terms coronary artery disease (CAD) or coronary vascular disease (CVD). All four terms can be used interchangeably, however we will predominately use ASCVD. A number of factors, such as high cholesterol and smoking, have been shown to be associated with increased risk of developing ASCVD.

Pathogenesis

Atherosclerotic plaques form primarily in the innermost lining of the artery, called the endothelium. The endothelium has several tasks and perhaps the most important is to prevent blood from forming clots inside the blood vessels.

Atherosclerosis begins with damage to the endothelium, such as mechanical trauma, and immunologic or chemical injury. A source of mechanical trauma is turbulent blood flow near areas where blood vessels branch off. The exact process by which damage occurs in humans has yet to be fully explained.

As a result, the platelets and clot-forming proteins in the blood form a small blood clot. After the clot has formed, over time, the body removes the blood clot and repairs the damage to the artery lining. Smooth muscle and other types of cells infiltrate the area of damage and are deposited to form an atherosclerotic plaque, or *atheroma*. This section of endothelium is prone to recurrent injury, and with each injury the atheroma grows thicker, blocking more of the artery.

The formation of atherosclerosis is a very gradual process, taking many years to progress to the point of causing symptoms. The process often begins when a person is in their 20s and 30s. The worsening blockage of an artery takes 20 or more years to develop.

Remember, atherosclerosis is the process that blocks the coronary arteries. The blockages can have several different effects on people, most commonly causing angina, a heart attack or sudden death. Although these three problems are related because atherosclerosis of the coronary arteries is their underlying cause, the problems affect a person's health in different ways.

Angina

The term angina (short for angina pectoris) refers to the chest pain that occurs when the heart is not receiving enough blood, usually because of partial blockages of one or more of the coronary arteries. Discomfort from heart injury feels different from other kinds of pain. While the heart has sensory nerves that can detect pain, these nerves are rudimentary and differ from the pain fibers found in our skin. As a result, the chest pain caused by ASCVD is typically described as a general chest "pressure," often radiating into the neck and arms. This poorly localized, vague pain is in direct contrast to the more sharp, well localized pain that occurs when the skin is injured.

The pain fibers in the heart are stimulated when the amount of oxygen getting to the heart is not adequate to meet the myocardium's need for oxygen. A typical scenario involves a coronary artery blockage that prevents an increase in blood flow to deliver more oxygen to the heart when it is working hard. For example, a man feels well at rest. However, when walking up a flight of stairs, he develops chest pressure. When he stops and rests, the "angina" gradually resolves. What has happened in this scenario is that our patient feels well at rest because the heart has adequate coronary artery blood flow. However, when he starts to exert his leg muscles by going up the stairs, the heart muscle is also working harder, and needs more oxygen. Unfortunately, the blockages in his coronary arteries limit the increase in blood flow to the heart muscle to deliver more oxygen. The heart muscle "downstream" from the blockages becomes *ischemic*, meaning that it has an inadequate amount of oxygen. The pain fibers in the ischemic myocardium are activated, causing chest pain. When he rests, the heart muscle is able to get adequate oxygen supply, and the chest pain gradually resolves.

Despite the chest pain, the heart muscle suffers no permanent damage if the ischemic condition does not last longer than a few minutes. When angina can be predictably brought on and relieved, as in the above scenario, it is called *stable* angina.

Unfortunately, angina is a poor warning signal (albeit an important one) that the coronary arteries have significant blockages. For unexplained reasons, roughly 25% of persons with heart disease do not feel the pain of angina, a phenomenon particularly common among diabetics. People with ASCVD can have episodes of myocardial ischemia and have no chest discomfort whatsoever. This condition is aptly called *silent ischemia* and medical science is wrestling with what this condition means for your health, and how to deal with it.

HEART ATTACK

A heart attack is one of the most common and most serious manifestations of ASCVD. Most heart attacks occur when a coronary artery is completely (or almost completely) occluded by a blood clot. In this instance, the blood clot grows into a large clot that completely blocks the coronary artery. This blockage can be further aggravated by the coronary artery narrowing in response to the blockage formation. This coronary artery "spasm" occurs in different degrees in different people. The heart muscle supplied by the occluded artery becomes ischemic, regardless of the workload of the heart, causing chest pain or angina. If blood flow is not reestablished in 10 to 15 minutes, heart muscle cells begin to die or infarct, resulting in a *myocardial infarction*.

The amount of heart muscle that dies depends on which coronary artery is blocked and where the blockage has occurred. The amount of damage to the heart can also be influenced by how well conditioned the heart is. Finally, reopening the occluded artery with "clot-dissolving" drugs or surgery at a hospital can decrease the size of the damage.

Normal functions of the heart are impaired when a portion of the myocardium dies. First, the efficiency of the heart decreases as the dead heart muscle is replaced by scar tissue that cannot contract. As a result of this decreased efficiency, the heart may not be able to pump an adequate supply of blood to the rest of the body. This condition is called *heart failure*. Many symptoms develop in heart failure, including shortness of breath, fatigue, and swelling of the lower legs. Until the scar tissue forms and strengthens (about six weeks) the heart wall is very weak in the area of the dead heart muscle cells. This area is prone to break open, or rupture, usually resulting in sudden death.

Sudden Death

A *sudden death* may be the first sign that someone has severe heart disease. The person suddenly (and literally) drops dead. The exact mechanism of death is not known for sure. Perhaps a blood clot forms in an area that results in massive damage. If the left main coronary artery becomes occluded, much of the heart's blood supply is blocked, and the heart quickly stops working. Sudden death can also result from serious abnormal heartbeats (arrhythmia). In both cases, the cessation of blood flow in the circulatory system results in unconsciousness within seconds and death within minutes.

Several other less common manifestations of ASCVD include passing out, abnormal shortness of breath, chronic fatigue, acute episodes of exhaustion, abnormal EKG, and abnormal heartbeats. Each of these can occur by themselves or in a variety of combinations.

DISEASES OF THE HEART MUSCLE (CARDIOMYOPATHY)

A number of conditions directly affect the heart muscle cells. These diseases of the myocardial cells are collectively called *cardiomyopathies*.

Dilated (or Congestive) Cardiomyopathy

Several diseases and chemicals can damage but not kill the heart muscle cells so that they do not contract normally. The myocardium becomes weak and "flabby." The result is a heart that enlarges (becomes dilated) and is much less efficient at pumping blood. Many times, the exact cause of an individual's cardiomyopathy goes undetected.

Viral infections, alcohol abuse, and chronic, uncontrolled hypertension are the most common causes of dilated cardiomyopathy. Occasionally, cases have been associated with either chronic or high level exposure to several elements, including arsenic, cobalt, lead, and antimony. Although fire fighters are not routinely exposed to these elements, certain groups of fire fighters may be exposed if working in industrial areas, which use these elements. Chronic exposure to low levels of organic solvents (such as toluene and trichloroethylene) can also cause cardiomyopathy. For fire fighters, exposure to these chemicals is also situational.

Cardiomyopathy has not been shown in any study to affect the health of fire fighters more than the rest of the population. Still, it is important to realize certain exposures can cause myocardial disease and that fire fighters may encounter those exposures.

Hypertrophic Cardiomyopathy

This group of diseases results from heart muscle cells actually growing. When this occurs, the muscle walls grow so thick that they actually block the heart valves, so blood cannot flow through the heart. The cause of this condition is unknown and has not been associated with any occupational exposures. There is a tendency for this problem to occur within families.

Restrictive Cardiomyopathy

This group of diseases is called *restrictive* because the heart muscle has difficulty relaxing, so that the heart has trouble refilling with blood. Unable to refill with blood, heart efficiency decreases. The heart cannot easily "relax" because various materials, such as a protein called amyloid, infiltrates and intermingles with the otherwise normal heart muscle cells, making the heart walls stiff. Most of the restrictive cardiomyopathies occur because of many different diseases like sarcoidosis, endocrine disorders, and certain cancers. Like hypertrophic cardiomyopathy, no clear occupational exposures are associated with the development of this disorder.

Left Ventricular Hypertrophy

Left ventricular hypertrophy (LVH) must be distinguished from hypertrophic cardiomyopathies. Hypertrophy refers to the growth and thickening of the heart muscle cells, but in this case it is in response to the heart having to work harder than normal. LVH most often develops in people with chronic, untreated high blood pressure. It occurs because the heart muscle, like any muscle in the body, bulks up (hypertrophies) when under heavy workloads. In this way, the heart muscle is no different than a muscle in the arm or leg of a weight lifter. Unfortunately, LVH predisposes the heart to many of the other diseases reviewed in this section.

DISEASES OF THE HEART VALVES

In most cases, valvular heart disease affects only one or two of the heart valves. Generally speaking, the left side of the heart (mitral and/or aortic valves) is more frequently affected. Most heart valve disease can be attributed to damage of the valve by infection (often by rheumatic fever) or congenital abnormalities. Years of constant opening and shutting cause small amounts of damage to progress into significant abnormalities.

The two most frequent valve problems are called stenosis and regurgitation. Stenosis means that the valve cannot open all the way, restricting blood flow through the heart. The heart must work harder to pump blood through these "narrowed" valves. Regurgitation means the valve leaks, so that blood flows the wrong way across the valve. This "backward" flow of blood results in the heart having to work harder, because it has to constantly "re-pump" a portion of the blood it just finished pumping. These valve conditions have characteristic heart "murmurs" that can be heard with a stethoscope. When either of these problems becomes severe enough to cause symptoms, open-heart surgery is typically done to replace the diseased valve. Increased risk of developing heart valve disease has not been associated with fire fighting, nor with any of the exposures fire fighters are likely to encounter.

Mitral Valve Prolapse

Mitral valve prolapse (MVP) refers to a largely genetic condition of the mitral valve that affects up to 10% of the population (primarily affecting women) of Canada and the United States. In MVP, the mitral valve leaflets are too long. The result is that the valve does not close properly. Instead of stopping shut in a normal position, the valves swing too far back, and "prolapse" into the left atrium. Although this condition can be associated with a heart murmur, atypical chest pains, and abnormal heartbeats, the vast majority of people with MVP have a normal life.

Infectious Endocarditis

Infectious endocarditis is the diagnosis given when certain microorganisms, such as bacteria, infect a heart valve. In addition to damaging the valve, infected valves frequently become covered with "blood clot–like" growths that can break off and travel through the arteries, eventually blocking an artery somewhere else in the body. Should the newly blocked artery be one that leads to the brain, a stroke may occur. Heart valves with previous damage from any cause are at increased likelihood to become infected. Although this is a relatively common diagnosis, no information suggests that fire fighters are at increased risk for this disease.

DISEASES OF THE CONDUCTION SYSTEM

As described earlier in this section, the conduction system consists of specialized heart cells that rapidly carry electric current through the heart, delivering the current to most all areas of the heart so that they contract together. This conduction system can have a large number of problems and abnormalities. The more serious problems are reviewed here.

Heart Block

The term *heart block* refers to electric signals not passing down the conduction system in a normal fashion. Blockages can be of varying degrees of severity, from a simple delay of the current to complete blockage. Complete blockage is called *complete heart block*, or *third-degree heart block*. This problem is analogous to cutting an electrical wire.

Third-degree heart block is the most dangerous type of heart block and usually results from damage to the conduction system during a heart attack. Lack of oxygen causes cells that make up the conduction system to die. Unfortunately, the cells most commonly affected are those in the AV node where the heart first receives electrical impulses to contract. Thus, when this critical area is damaged, no current enters the ventricles and they stop working.

To treat this condition, doctors can implant artificial pacemakers. Pacemakers are small, battery-driven devices that deliver electric shocks to the myocardium in the ventricles, causing them to contract normally.

Arrhythmias

The term *arrhythmia* refers to abnormal heartbeats. Arrhythmias occur because the normal, orderly delivery and movement of the electric current in the heart is disrupted, resulting from ischemia, scar tissue, cardiomyopathies, and valve problems.

When electric current is completely erratic in the atria, small areas of the atria contract haphazardly. This condition is called *atrial fibrillation*. This type of contraction does not generate enough force to pump any blood. However, as the atria are not essential for the ventricles to fill, most people do well with atrial fibrillation. This can usually be controlled with medication.

The same erratic current can occur in the ventricles, and is called *ventricular fibrillation*. Because the ventricles do not pump any blood during fibrillation, there is rapid loss of consciousness and death. The treatment is to "cardiovert" the heart by delivering a large electric shock to the heart. This shock can cancel the erratic current in the heart, allowing the normal heart beat mechanism to take over.

Ventricular tachycardia is another dangerous arrhythmia. The ventricles develop a rapid heartbeat (150 to 300 beats per minute), in which electric currents bypass the normal heart conduction system. In addition to the rapid heartbeat, the heart muscle contraction is less coordinated than normal. The resulting rapid, inefficient pumping of the heart can result in a low blood pressure that requires emergency medical treatment.

A number of chemicals have been shown to "sensitize" the myocardium, making the development of arrhythmias from irritations of the myocardium more likely. This is particularly worrisome in people who already have underlying heart disease. These include halogenated hydrocarbons, organophosphates, antimony, arsenic and arsine. Although exposure to these chemicals will be highly situational for fire fighters, the increasing use of synthetic polymers and chemicals increases the potential for exposure, especially to halogenated hydrocarbons.

FIRE FIGHTER RISK FACTORS

This section reviews occupational exposures faced by fire fighters that may increase the risk of developing atherosclerotic plaques or may precipitate a heart attack in fire fighters with underlying ASCVD.

CARBON MONOXIDE

Carbon monoxide (CO) is formed by the incomplete combustion of carbon-containing materials. Personal monitors worn by fire fighters have recorded very high concentrations of CO at fires. Carbon monoxide decreases the oxygen carrying ability of the blood and poses acute and chronic health effects.

Carbon monoxide acts as a chemical asphyxiant and starves the heart of its normal oxygen supply by binding to the oxygen-carrying molecule, hemoglobin. Carbon monoxide binds to hemoglobin 200 times more effectively than oxygen, so it takes only a small percentage of CO in the inspired air for hemoglobin molecules to become filled with CO. Once bound to hemoglobin, it is difficult to remove CO from the oxygen-binding site. The net effect is that even low concentrations of CO in the air can have significant negative effects on the body's ability to transport oxygen.

At high CO exposure levels, the oxygen-carrying capacity of blood becomes compromised and the death of myocardium (similar to a heart attack) can occur, even without any blockages in the coronary arteries. The physical demands of fire fighting increase the body's demand for oxygen and can worsen symptoms. High level of exposure can also result in loss of consciousness due to lack of oxygen sent to the brain. In persons with known ASCVD accompanied by angina, CO exposure has been shown to reduce exercise capacity and result in vulnerability to cardiac rhythm disturbances.

The reduced capability of the blood to carry oxygen following CO exposure functionally worsens existing heart artery blockages, resulting in decreased oxygen delivery to heart muscle. Reduced exercise capacity and ischemic responses have also been shown in healthy young adults exposed to CO. Long-term exposure to CO is suspected to cause the formation of atherosclerotic plaques.

Since the only significant entryway for CO into the body is through the lungs, fire fighters can protect themselves from excessive exposure by proper use of personal protective equipment, such as the self-contained breathing apparatus.

POLYCYCLIC AROMATIC HYDROCARBONS

Polycyclic aromatic hydrocarbons (PAHs) are a group of carbon compounds that are formed in most fires involving carbon-containing materials, including wood, fuels and many man-made materials. Like carbon monoxide, studies of long-term exposure to PAHs have shown an accelerated formation of atherosclerotic plaques in animals. However, this association has never been clearly demonstrated in people. Unlike CO, PAHs are not asphyxiants. However, they are considered carcinogens in the lungs and colon.

OTHER CHEMICALS

A number of other chemicals that can be present in combustion products can have adverse effects on the heart. Cyanide and hydrogen sulfide act as chemical asphyxiants, potentially resulting in myocardial ischemia. Arsenic and carbon disulfide exposure may contribute to atherosclerotic plaque formation. Lead, cadmium, and organic solvent exposure may contribute to the development of high blood pressure, thus indirectly affecting the heart. The potential for exposure to these dangerous chemicals increases as the normal industrial mechanisms used to control exposure fail during fire and disaster situations.

OCCUPATIONAL STRESS

A number of studies have demonstrated that fire fighters suffer from increased psychological stress. The psychological stress accompanying alarm response is frequently accompanied by physical changes. For example, the heart rate of fire fighters has been found to markedly increase – an average of 47 to 61 beats per minute – when a fire alarm sounds, and the heart rate will remain elevated until arrival at the fire scene, despite minimal physical exertion. The level to which stress increases heart disease risk has yet to be accurately determined, but may be small relative to other risk factors.

NOISE

Noise is a physical stressor that is known to cause the release of adrenaline, resulting in increased blood pressure. The characteristics of the noise that have been associated with heart disease include unpredictability, a lack of meaningfulness, high volume, and of an intermittent nature. Studies of fire fighters' reaction to alarm signals have confirmed that noise can induce measurable biologic and psychological effects. Heart rates, particularly among younger fire fighters, increase to as much as 130 to150 beats per minute after exposure to the station fire alarm. Several additional studies have demonstrated 47 to 61 beat-per-minute increases after exposure to alarms. It has been theorized that these responses result from release of catecholamines, including adrenaline. A theorized disruptor to the endothelium could be a contributing factor to the increased risk of heart disease among fire fighters.

Further evidence is provided by a NIOSH study performed in conjunction with Raytheon. The medical records of factory workers regularly exposed to noise levels of 95 dB or greater were compared to workers exposed at 80 dB or less. The findings showed a statistically significant increase in the number of cardiovascular diseases in the high exposure group. Thus, loud noise exposure appears to result in a small, but measurable, increase in heart disease risk.

One possible solution to address this situation is to modify existing alarm systems so that alarms sound only in stations that are required to respond. To minimize the impact on hearing and the cardiovascular system, they should ring with a gradually increasing volume rather than at full volume from the outset.

HEAT AND COLD

Both excessive heat and excessive cold have been linked to an increased risk of heart attack, especially in those persons with existing coronary artery blockages. Cold causes blood vessels to constrict, elevating blood pressure, thereby increasing how hard the heart must work. Heat increases the heart's workload, as it must pump more blood to the skin as the body tries to cool itself. Either stress can presumably induce a heart attack if demands on the heart are excessive.

PREVENTING HEART DISEASE

There are a number of important lifestyle and health-related factors that are of great importance in determining your risk of heart disease. These modifiable risk factors include: smoking, hypertension, high blood cholesterol (hypercholesterolemia), diabetes, and obesity. These risk factors become more important as we age and heart disease becomes more common. While aging is not reversible, the lifestyle choices that we make are and can dramatically reduce the risk of ASCVD. If you have already been diagnosed with hypertension, diabetes, or elevated cholesterol, the treatment plan recommended by your physician, coupled with the choices that you make, provide a comprehensive strategy to reduce your risk of heart disease. These important choices include: tobacco use, exercise, weight control, and stress management. In this section we will discuss ideas that will assist you in making and maintaining heart healthy choices.

SMOKING CESSATION

CIGARETTES AND OTHER FORMS OF TOBACCO ARE ADDICTIVE. Physically, nicotine's addictive nature is due to its stimulation of the brain and heart. Psychologically, cigarette use is reinforced by specific activities and social interaction. We may use cigarettes as a reward after persevering through stressful situations, or as a means to strike up a conversation. Given these facts, it is no surprise that so many people have been unsuccessful in the attempt to "kick the habit." In fact, most persons who quit for good are able to do so only after multiple attempts. Fortunately, there are millions of former smokers who have successfully beaten the habit, and can attest to the fact that their lives are just as happy and fulfilling, or even more so, without smoking. In consideration of the ill health effects associated with tobacco use, the IAFF has proposed three main goals in its Wellness-Fitness Initiative Tobacco Cessation Policy:

1. All new fire department candidates shall be tobacco free upon appointment and throughout their length of service to the department.

2. Current fire department uniformed personnel shall not use tobacco products inside the work-site, within or on fire department apparatus, or inside training facilities.

3. A fire department sanctioned tobacco cessation program shall be made available to incumbent tobacco users. Tobacco cessation programs must be non-punitive and must include short- and long-term goals.

The Wellness-Fitness Initiative also describes examples of tobacco cessation programs. The IAFF has also published *The IAFF Smoking Cessation Manual: Issues, Policies, and Programs* to assist you in your smoking cessation efforts. It outlines the most commonly used techniques, including aversive therapy, self-help and group programs, nicotine replacement (with "patches" or "gum"), acupuncture, and other methods. No single method is right for everyone. But, regardless of which method you choose, several decisions will increase your success rate.

STEPS YOU CAN TAKE TODAY

- Contact the IAFF for a copy of the smoking cessation manual.

- Consider using nicotine replacement therapy, such as "the patch" or "nicotine gum," regardless of which group or self-help method you choose. When used in a comprehensive program, nicotine replacement roughly doubles the success rate.

If you desire additional information on individual programs or your department wishes to begin a smoking cessation program, contact the IAFF Department of Occupational Health and Safety.

IAFF POLICY

Over the past several years the issue of infectious (communicable) disease in the fire service has taken on a new and urgent meaning with the advent of AIDS, hepatitis, and tuberculosis. However, the range of diseases that may affect fire fighters, EMTs, and paramedics goes well beyond this list. The IAFF *1998 Death and Injury Survey* reports that 1 out of every 32 fire fighters was exposed to tuberculosis, 5.8% were exposed to hepatitis B, 6.5% were exposed to hepatitis C, 14.6% were exposed to human immunodeficiency virus, and 43.3% were exposed to some other communicable disease.

The goal of the section is to provide a background in the nature of the infections of concern to fire fighters and how they are recognized and prevented.

Infectious disease is an area of rapidly changing conditions. Some of the controversies that may be expected in the next several years include the issue of baseline screening for hepatitis B and C, mandatory testing for HIV, and whether to regulate exposures for non-bloodborne pathogens such as tuberculosis. While this manual may discuss some of these issues, this will continue to be an evolving field.

Through the Wellness-Fitness Initiative and NFPA 1500, fire departments are responsible for evaluating the health status of all fire fighters, EMTs, and paramedics and their ability to perform assigned duties.

All fire departments must adopt NFPA 1500, especially in light of federal and state requirements for implementing fire department infection control programs. Such programs must include policy guidelines for the prevention of transmission of bloodborne pathogens and other infectious diseases during fire fighter, EMT, and paramedic response activities as well as guidelines for improving infection control practices. The fire department must be responsible for providing barrier protection equipment (e.g., gloves, protective garments), safer needle devices, supplies, proper disinfection facilities, and appropriate training.

The fire department must implement annual training for all fire department personnel in universal blood and body fluid precautions, barrier techniques, safer needle devices, and other scientifically accepted infection control policies. Such training also should provide information on infectious disease risk factors and the contagiousness and transmission of infectious disease as well as information on the availability and merits of voluntary, confidential or anonymous counseling and testing as a personal health measure for fire department personnel. Training materials must include information on exposure to infectious diseases and reproductive health.

The fire department must establish procedures for the evaluation of work limitations for employees with an infectious disease who in the course of performing their duties demonstrate evidence of functional impairment or inability to adhere to standard infection control practices or who present an excessive risk of infection to patients or fire department members. The fire department physician must evaluate fire fighter, EMT, and paramedic job duties to determine job limitations, if any, in the event of an individual's infectious disease. The evaluation should include an assessment of any factors that may compromise the performance of job duties, as well as a review of scientifically and medically accepted infection control practices. Factors include illness or presence of exudative or weeping lesions that may interfere significantly with the fire fighters', EMTs', and paramedics' ability to perform their jobs and provide quality care. Both physical and mental competencies are also to be considered. Additionally, the fire department physician should review the immunologic status of the fire fighter, EMT, and paramedic and susceptibility to infectious diseases.

The fire department physician must assist with developing policies addressing limited duty assignment for non-infectious personnel where there is a greater potential for that individual to contract an infectious disease. Fire fighters, EMTs, and paramedics with extensive skin lesions or severe dermatitis on hands, arms, head, face, or neck must be evaluated to determine whether they should engage in direct patient contact, handle patient care equipment, or handle medical waste until such time that they are healed.

INFECTIOUS DISEASES OF CONCERN TO FIRE FIGHTERS

Occupational contagious diseases are infectious diseases that are contracted through the course of a person performing his or her work. These contagious diseases are usually caused by viruses or bacteria, though in some occupations parasitic agents are important. Occupationally contracted contagious diseases are considered compensable through the workers' compensation system, just like any other occupationally caused disease. The infectious diseases of primary concern to fire fighters include hepatitis B virus (HBV); hepatitis C virus (HCV); human immunodeficiency virus (HIV), which is the viral agent responsible for causing the acquired immunodeficiency syndrome (AIDS); and tuberculosis (TB). Other infectious diseases of importance to fire fighters, although not as occupationally common, include the hepatitis viruses A, D, and E, herpes, influenza, lyme disease, meningitis, mumps, scabies, and tetanus.

While working, fire fighters often respond to emergency situations involving victims who have been injured and are actively bleeding. The victim may require extrication from a difficult-to-access accident scene, such as a motor vehicle accident or poorly accessible building. There may be broken glass or other sharp objects at the scene that are poorly visualized, and the lighting at the scene may be minimal. In addition, if the victim is hemorrhaging and needs to be extricated quickly to save his/her life, the emergency provider may act in haste, with disregard for his or her own safety. Fire fighters also may be involved in emergency medical treatment at the scene, including intravenous line insertion and blood drawing. The fire fighter almost never knows the infectious disease status of the victim while he or she is rendering emergency services. All of these factors combine to place the fire fighter at increased risk of contracting a bloodborne contagious disease through a puncture wound, skin abrasion, or laceration that can become contaminated with infected blood or other potentially infectious material.

Education and training are the most effective means available to limit the risk of contracting a bloodborne contagious disease in fire fighters. The risk of contracting an infectious disease, and methods used to avoid exposure, should be a part of every fire fighter's education. Universal precautions, such as the wearing of protective gloves, safety glasses, masks, and gowns, should be used whenever exposure to blood and/or other bodily fluids is possible. These precautions should be taken whether or not the infectious status of the patient is known.

The regulations outlined by the Occupational Safety and Health Administration (OSHA) outlined in 29 CFR 1910.1030, *Bloodborne Pathogens*, require any personnel who are potentially exposed to bloodborne pathogens to be equipped with personal protective equipment sufficient to prevent such exposures.

The few seconds that it takes for the fire fighter to don protective gear in order to protect himself or herself will not make a significant difference in the survival of the patient. Fire fighters should be trained to automatically don protective gear, to carefully evaluate possible hazards at the scene that may cause lacerations or abrasions, and to maximize the lighting available at the scene as much as possible to better visualize the hazards.

APPLICABLE REGULATIONS AND STANDARDS

OSHA STANDARD ON BLOODBORNE PATHOGENS

On December 2, 1991, the Occupational Safety and Health Administration promulgated a new standard for bloodborne pathogens that greatly changed how fire fighters, emergency response personnel, and all other workers potentially exposed to bloodborne diseases should be trained and equipped to protect themselves from infections. The standard, which is known as the Bloodborne Pathogens standard (29 CFR 1910.1030) was published in the Federal Register on December 6, 1991 (56 FR 64004) and was revised on November 5, 1999 (CPL 2-2.44D).

NFPA 1500 REQUIREMENTS

The NFPA 1500, *Standard on Fire Department Occupational Safety and Health Program*, was developed to provide a consensus standard for an occupational safety and health program for the fire service. The intent of this standard is to provide the framework for a safety and health program for a fire department or any type of organization providing similar services.

NFPA 1581 REQUIREMENTS

The NFPA 1581, *Standard on Fire Department Infection Control Program* (2000), addresses the provision of minimum requirements for infection control practices within a fire department. The purpose of the standard is *"to provide minimum criteria for infection control in the fire station, in the fire apparatus and during procedures at an incident scene, and at any other area where fire department members are involved in routine or emergency operations."*(1-2.1)

REFERENCES

American Cancer Society. (1993). *Facts on Skin Cancer*. Pub. 88-400M-Rev. 5/93-No. 2049.

Atlas, E.L. et al. (1985). Chemical and biological characterization of emissions for a fireperson training facility. *American Industrial Hygiene Association Journal*, 46, 532–540.

Barnard, R.J. & Weber, J.S. (1979). Carbon monoxide: a hazard to fire fighters. *Archives of Environmental Health*, 34, 255–257.

Bhatia, R. et al. (1998). Diesel exhaust exposure and lung cancer. *Epidemiology*, 9, 84–91.

Bizovi, K.E. & Leikin, J.D. (1995). Smoke inhalation among firefighters. *Occupational Medicine: State of the Art Reviews*, 10, 4, 721–733.

Burgess, W.A. et al. (1999). Minimum protection factors for respiratory protective devices for firefighters. *American Industrial Hygiene Association Journal*, 38, 18–23.

Centers for Disease Control and Prevention. (1990). *The Health Benefits of Smoking Cessation*. Department of Health and Human Services, Publication No. (CDC) 90-8416.

Doll, R. & Peto, R. (1981). The causes of cancer: quantitative estimated of avoidable risks of cancer in the United States today. *Journal of the National Cancer Institute*, 66, 1191–1308.

Froines, J.R. et al. (1987). Exposure of fire fighters to diesel emissions in fire stations. *American Industrial Hygiene Association Journal*, 48, 202–207.

Garshick, E. et al. (1988). A retrospective cohort study of lung cancer and diesel exhaust exposure in railroad workers. *American Review of Respiratory Disorders*, 137, 4, 820–825.

Girod G. (1990). *Station Pollution: Lungs at Risk*. The California Fire Service, Nov.

Golden, A. et al. (1995). The risk of cancer in firefighters. *Occupational Medicine: State of the Art Reviews*, 10, 4, 803–820.

Guidotti, T.L. (1998). Applying epidemiology to adjudication. *Occupational Medicine: State of the Art Reviews*, 13, 2.

Guidotti, T.L. & Clough, V.M. (1992). Occupational health concerns of firefighting. *Annual Review of Public Health*, 13, 151–171.

Gustavsson, P. et al. (1998). Occupational exposures and squamous cell carcinoma of the oral cavity, pharynx, larynx, and oesaphagus: a case-control study in Sweden. *Journal of Occupational and Environmental Medicine*, 55, 393–400.

Hausen, H. Z. (1991). Viruses in human cancer. *Science*, 254, 1167.

Henriks-Eckerman, M. et al. (1990). Thermal degradation products of steel protective paints. *American Industrial Hygiene Association Journal*, 51, 241–244.

International Agency for Research on Cancer. (1989). *Monographs on the evaluation of the carcinogenic risks to humans: Diesel and gasoline engine exhausts and some nitroarenes*. Lyon, France 46, 148–154.

Karstadt, M. (1998). Availability of epidemiologic data for chemicals known to cause cancer in animals: an update. *American Journal of Industrial Medicine*, 34, 519–525.

Lees, P.S.J. (1995). Combustion products and other firefighter exposures. *Occupational Medicine: State of the Art Reviews*, 10, 691–706.

Lowry, W.T. et al. (1985). Studies of toxic gas production during actual structural fires in the Dallas area. *Journal of Forensic Science*, 30, 59–72.

McDiarmid, M.A. et al. (1991). Reproductive hazards of fire fighting II: Chemical hazards. *American Journal of Industrial Medicine*, 19, 447–472.

Rom, W.N., ed. (1998). *Environmental and Occupational Medicine*. Philadelphia: Lippincott-Raven.

Siemiatycki, J. (1991). *Risk Factors for Cancer in the Workplace*. Boca Raton, Fla.: CRC Press.

Steenland, K. et al. (1996). Review of occupational lung carcinogens. *American Journal of Industrial Medicine*, 29, 5, 474–490.

Talaska, G. et al. (1996). Polycyclic aromatic hydrocarbons (PAHs), Nitro-PAHs and related environmental compounds: Biological markers of exposure and effects. *Environmental Health Perspectives*, 104, 901–906.

U.S. Department of Health and Human Services: National Center for Health Statistics. (1999). *National Vital Statistics Reports: Births and Deaths, preliminary data for July 1997 to June 1998*, DHHS Publication No (PHS) 99-1120, 9-0472, June.

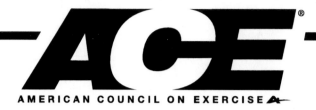

AMERICAN COUNCIL ON EXERCISE

If you would like to receive information about the following ACE products and services, please contact our Customer Service department at (800) 825-3636, Ext. 653.

- ◆ Other ACE certifications and programs:
  - • Group Fitness Instructor
  - • Personal Trainer
  - • Clinical Exercise Specialist
  - • Lifestyle & Weight Management Consultant
- ◆ Additional resource materials (e.g., books, videos)
- ◆ The Fire FitKids community outreach program
- ◆ Serving as a host site for the Peer Fitness Trainer exam

Also, visit the ACE Web site at www.acefitness.org to receive additional information about the Peer Fitness Trainer Certification.

- ◆ Tips for passing the Peer Fitness Trainer certification exam
- ◆ The complete Exam Content Outline, which outlines the topics covered on the exam, helping you to better focus your studies